ILLUSTRATED ELEMENTS OF

ALEXANDER
TECHNIQUE

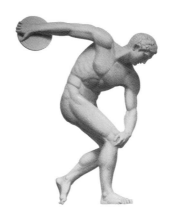

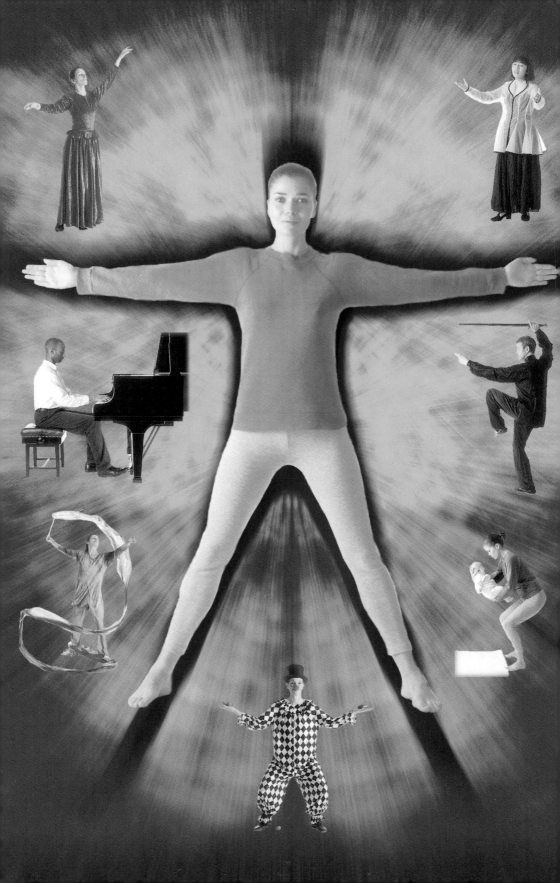

ILLUSTRATED ELEMENTS OF
ALEXANDER TECHNIQUE

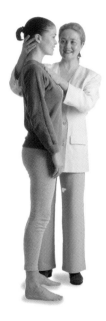

GLYNN MACDONALD

ELEMENT

First published in 2002 by Element
An Imprint of HarperCollins*Publishers*
77–85 Fulham Palace Road
Hammersmith, London W6 8JB

ELEMENT™ is a trademark of HarperCollins*Publishers* Ltd

2 4 6 8 10 9 7 5 3 1

Text copyright © Glynn Macdonald 2002
Copyright © HarperCollins*Publishers* 2002

Glynn Macdonald asserts the moral right
to be identified as the author of this work

This book was created by THE BRIDGEWATER BOOK COMPANY

A catalogue record of this book
is available from the British Library

ISBN 0 00 713385 5

Printed and bound in Hong Kong by Printing Express

NOTE FROM PUBLISHER
Any information given in this book is not intended to be taken as a
replacement for medical advice. Any person with a condition requiring
medical attention should consult a qualified practitioner or therapist.

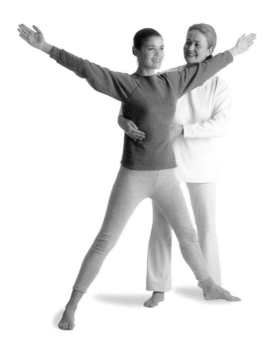

Contents

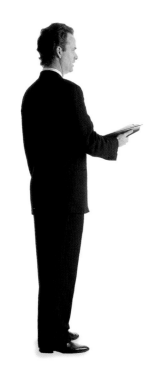

Know Thyself

Know then thyself, presume not God to scan;
The proper study of mankind is Man.
Placed on this isthmus of a middle state,
A being darkly wise and rudely great:
With too much knowledge for the Sceptic side,
With too much weakness for the Stoic's pride,
He hangs between; in doubt to act or rest,
In doubt to deem himself a God or Beast,
In doubt his mind or body to prefer;
Born but to die, and reasoning but to err;
Alike in ignorance, his reason such
Whether he thinks too little or too much:
Chaos of thought and passion, all confused;
Still by himself abused, or disabused;
Created half to rise and half to fall;
Great lord of all things, yet a prey to all;
Sole judge of truth, in endless error hurled:
The glory, jest, and riddle of the world!

ALEXANDER POPE (1688–1744)

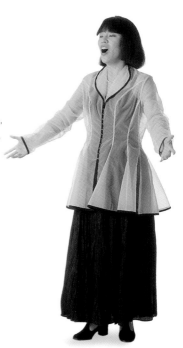

Introduction

THE ALEXANDER TECHNIQUE *is a method for organizing both your sensations and intentions of movement, where you are in space and in time, by becoming more conscious of your mind and body, and the world around you. Conscious guidance and control offer you the possibility to experience more unity and ease in everyday activities. The Alexander Technique, tested and proved in all walks of life in the last 100 years, recognizes that*

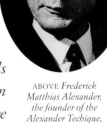

ABOVE *Frederick Matthias Alexander, the founder of the Alexander Techique, was born in 1869.*

any action we perform depends for its efficiency and success on how well the mind and body are functioning in unison.

> Each waking day is a stage dominated for good or ill, in comedy, farce, or tragedy by a "dramatis person," the self, and so it will be until the curtain drops. The self is a unity… it regards itself as one, others treat it as one, the logic of grammar endorses this by a pronoun in the singular. All its diversity is merged in oneness.
>
> **CHARLES SHERRINGTON**

We can recognize someone who is depressed by how they stand, sit, and walk. The joy of a child who is taking its first steps is equally apparent. We can re-learn this unconscious joy. As we become more "in touch" with ourselves, our knowledge and understanding of ourselves increases.

The Alexander Technique coordinates mind and body in all activities of living. In the process it organizes our sensations of movement, our feelings and emotions, and our experiences of the world around us. It helps us to be conscious of both our "internal" and "external" world. It allows us to be present with all our being. When you have conscious control, you can become an originator of life. As you release undue tension, you will release the creativity you possess. You can begin to live in the here and now, conscious of what you are doing, what you are

LEFT *A journey of 1,000 miles starts with the first step. The joy of a child's first step is universally shared.*

feeling, and with the power to bring about change in yourself and your life.

How to Use this Book

The Alexander Technique is often characterized as a kind of physical control drill consisting of a series of rules and regulations – sit up straight, do not slouch, do not cross your legs. Nothing could be further from the truth. *Illustrated Elements of Alexander Technique* brings together the collective experience of practitioners of the Technique from all over the world to give a fascinating and inspiring picture of this educational therapy. It is not a rulebook; rather it is a program for releasing unnecessary tension and accumulated bad postural habits, encouraging your own self-awareness, and giving conscious control back to the full person.

BELOW **The next section describes the basic principles of good use, looking at the way unconscious behavior limits our bodies' natural ability to function efficiently.**

BELOW **The first part of the book gives an account of the history and development of the Technique, and the scientific basis for F.M. Alexander's original discoveries.**

Lists of do's and don'ts help you to observe, identify, and eradicate bad habits.

Detailed artwork illustrates the basic anatomical principles that underpin Alexander's theories.

Step-by-step sequences use clear photographs to demonstrate good posture.

BELOW **Drawing on examples from the performing arts, sports, and everyday activities, the Alexander Technique is shown in action.**

Individual case studies draw on the actual experiences of Alexander teachers and practitioners to explain the ways in which the Technique helped with many specific problems.

Various problems, with posture and bad patterns, are exemplified and explained with photographs.

7

Historical Background and Biography

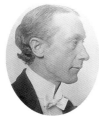

FREDERICK MATTHIAS ALEXANDER – *the founder of the Alexander Technique – was born in Australia on January 20, 1869. He came from a family that had succeeded in making a life for themselves in a remote outpost on the island of Tasmania, south of the mainland. His background and upbringing made him naturally observant, self-reliant, and disciplined. From his early youth, one of his chief pleasures was studying the plays of Shakespeare.*

Alexander became interested in the art of reciting and decided to take it up as a profession, concentrating especially on the great speeches from Shakespeare. In the middle of the last century, electronic amplification did not exist, so performers had to rely solely on the strength of their natural vocal ability to project their voices. In trying to satisfy the demands that Shakespearean text put upon him as a performer, Alexander began to have trouble with his throat, which affected his voice. He could not control the problem, and at times he lost his voice completely, a medical condition known as aphonia.

He consulted doctors and voice trainers, and the medical diagnosis given to him was irritation of the mucous membrane of the throat and nose with inflammation of the vocal cords. The medical advice was that he should rest his voice and speak as little as possible between performances. He followed this advice, but by the time he came to the end of his next recital he could hardly

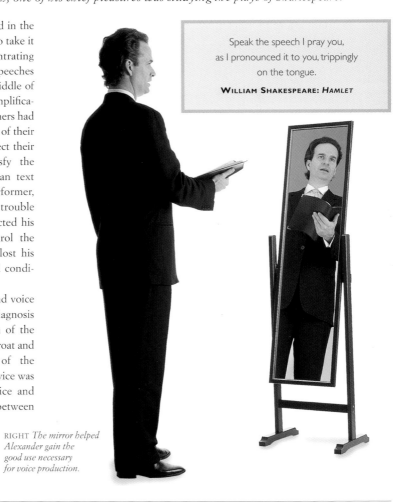

Speak the speech I pray you,
as I pronounced it to you, trippingly
on the tongue.

WILLIAM SHAKESPEARE: HAMLET

RIGHT *The mirror helped Alexander gain the good use necessary for voice production.*

speak, and it seemed as though his chosen career had come to an end. His doctor suggested that he continue with the resting treatment, but Alexander argued that he could not go along with this; he had followed advice to rest and his voice had been fine, but after only an hour of performing the symptoms had returned, and were just as bad as they were before. He asked the doctor whether it was not fair to conclude that it was something he was doing in using his voice that was causing the trouble. The doctor agreed, but could not suggest what that something might be. Alexander resolved that he must try to find out for himself.

EARLY EXPERIMENTS

Alexander decided to use a mirror to give him feedback and help him see what he was doing while speaking the text. He realized that he was continually pulling his head backward when he came to speak. He also observed that he was lifting his chest, arching his spine, narrowing his lower back, stiffening his legs, and pushing his toes into the floor as well as retracting his head, which was the determining factor in reducing the efficiency of his voice. He said: "I had to admit that I had never thought out how I directed the use of myself, but that I had used myself habitually in the way that felt natural to me."

The mirror reflected movements of which he was unaware. In his book, *The Use of the Self*, he says:

I refused to believe that problem was hopeless... "Surely," I argued, "if it is possible for feeling to be untrustworthy as a means of direction, it should be possible to make it trustworthy again." Shakespeare's idea of the wonderful potentialities of man had long been a source of inspiration to me: "What a piece of work is a man! How noble in reason! How infinite in faculties! In form and moving, how express and admirable! In action, how like an angel! In apprehension how like a god!"

LET THE HEAD GO FORWARD AND UP

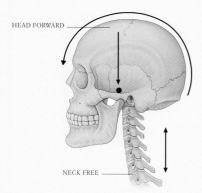

HEAD FORWARD

NECK FREE

Because the majority of the weight of the skull is in front of the spine, the head is naturally inclined to nod forward effortlessly. This allows the neck pressure to be released.

For use oft changes
the very stamp of nature.

WILLIAM SHAKESPEARE: *HAMLET*

LET THE SPINE LENGTHEN

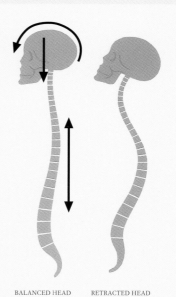

BALANCED HEAD   RETRACTED HEAD

When the head is pulled back and down (retracted), the spine cannot achieve its full length. When the head is freely balanced in the same direction as the center of gravity, the neck and spine can lengthen.

CONSCIOUS INHIBITION AND CONSCIOUS DIRECTION

Spurred on by the possibility of fulfilling his potential, Alexander continued his experimental work on himself in front of the mirror. Each time he saw he was interfering with his good posture, he would patiently stop. The nature of the control is indirect. If the head is correctly balanced on the body, breathing takes care of itself. In order to achieve this balance, Alexander realized that, first of all, the misuse had to be stopped so he could proceed in a new direction – allowing the neck to be free so that the head could go forward and up, and the back could

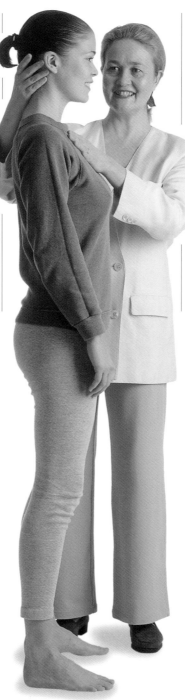

Let the head go forward and up. The gentle hands of the teacher prevent the pupil from pulling her head back and down and restricting her breathing.

Let the back lengthen and widen. The pupil begins to stand in a balanced way, at her full height.

lengthen and widen. These directions changed the whole use of the body, leading to improved functioning.

These directions are only possible if the inhibitory process is set in place to start with (see Conscious Inhibition page 23). Inhibition is the key to conscious control of direction. He needed to stop for a second and detach himself from the stiffening and contracting that was occurring inside him. When he calmed down the unnecessary internal activity, then he could stop holding his breath and objectively decide not to react mindlessly. This allows the level of tension that often precedes any action to be reduced. Alexander

Let the breath return freely. The hands of the teacher remind the pupil not to collapse down in front as she breathes out.

LEFT *Alexander Technique teachers help their pupils to experience Conscious Inhibition and Direction.*

> Release me from my bands with
> the help of your good hands.
>
> **WILLIAM SHAKESPEARE:**
> **THE TEMPEST**

had discovered that if he could stop the wrong habits, then the right direction could happen.

Gradually he began to develop an understanding of how his head, neck, and back could work harmoniously together and in what ways he was interfering with that optimum functioning. The inflammation of the vocal cords disappeared and his voice became reliable and effective. His general health also improved. By an indirect route Alexander had made a significant scientific discovery. Professor John Dewey said in his Introduction to *The Use of the Self*:

I cannot speak with too much admiration of the persistence and thoroughness with which these extremely difficult experiments and observations were carried out. In consequence, Mr. Alexander created what may be truly called a physiology of the living organism.

The sucking and gasping for air which had so bothered him stopped, and his breathing improved greatly. He then realized that imperfect breathing was not limited to those with vocal problems but applied to most people. Our breathing patterns give a very true indication of both our physical and emotional states.

THE ART OF BREATHING

In the 19th century, consumption, also known as respiratory tuberculosis, was the single most common cause of death. Rising living standards and improved hygiene made the incidence of the disease decrease, but at the turn of the century the only treatment available was rest, good diet, and as much fresh air as possible. In 1903, Alexander wrote an article entitled, "The Prevention and Cure of Consumption," in which he described his "art of breathing," listing the following benefits from the practice of his Technique:

Lungs
1 A far greater quantity of air is inspired into and expelled from the lungs.

Oxygenation
2 The oxygenation of the blood is more adequate.

"Vital Capacity"
3 The "vital capacity" is greater and easily available.

Thorax
4 The mobility of the thorax is increased daily.

Lung Tissue
5 The lung tissue is nourished in much greater degree.

Digestion
6 Stimulation of the digestive organs increases.

Respiration
7 The strain in respiration and speaking is removed from the throat.

Breathing
8 Nasal breathing (night and day) is firmly established.

Heart
9 The heart's action is improved daily.

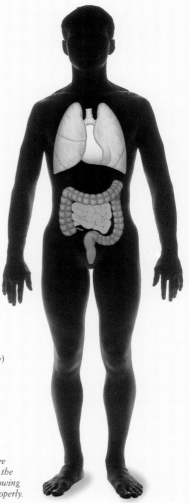

RIGHT *Good posture relieves pressure on the internal organs, allowing them to function properly.*

Scientific Verification

FROM THE BEGINNING *doctors and scientists realized that Alexander had discovered a fundamental principle in human movement and behavior. During his lifetime several doctors testified to the effects of his technique in medical journals. In 1937, 19 doctors urged in a letter in the* British Medical Journal *that the Alexander Technique should be included in medical training.*

One of the fundamental principles of the Alexander Technique is that use affects functioning – that is – the way we "use" ourselves (move, think, etc.) affects how well we function. A second principle is that the organism functions as a whole. So the execution of a specific movement reflects the overall functioning of the organism. As Sir Charles Sherrington confirmed in *The Endeavour of Jean Fernel*:

> *Mr. Alexander has done a service to the subject by insistently treating each act as involving the whole integrated individual, the whole psychophysical man. To take a step is an affair, not of this or that limb solely, but of the total neuromuscular activity of the moment – not least of the head and neck.*

A third principle of the Technique states that the relationship between the head, neck, and back has a paramount influence on the whole organism, its posture and health. Scientific support for this contention came in the 1920s with the publication of Professor Magnus' experiments with animals, which suggested that the head-neck-back relationship had a dominating influence on the position and attitude of the rest of the body.

Eminent scientists have testified to Alexander's scientific method and results. Raymond Dart, the famous anthropologist, wrote in his book *Skill and Poise* that:

Electronic facilities have confirmed Alexander's insights and authenticated the Technique he discovered in the 1890s of teaching both average and skilled adult individuals to become aware of their wrong body

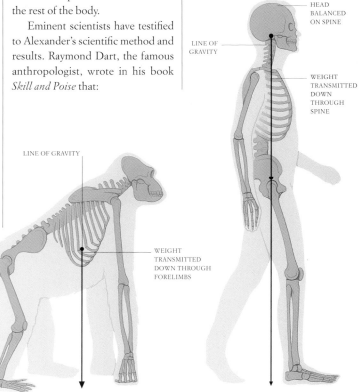

HEAD BALANCED ON SPINE

LINE OF GRAVITY

WEIGHT TRANSMITTED DOWN THROUGH SPINE

LINE OF GRAVITY

WEIGHT TRANSMITTED DOWN THROUGH FORELIMBS

RIGHT *The relative positions of the head and the body, and the different parts of the body to the head and neck, exercise a profound and important influence both on the bodily coordination and on the muscles actually concerned.*

use, how to eliminate handicaps and thus achieve better (i.e. increasingly skilled) use of themselves, both physically and mentally.

Dr. T. D. M. Roberts researching at the University of Glasgow found "If this awareness can be achieved, the patient's posture thereafter becomes more supple and consequently more comfortable to maintain."

Dr. David Garlick who heads the Laboratory for Muscolosketeral and Postural Research in the University of New South Wales has found "A person's usual sitting or standing posture will be accepted at a subconscious level as appropriate or normal even though, in extreme cases, knees are hyperextended, lumber lordosis is accentuated, thoracic curve is exaggerated. The human cerebellum appears to have a posture pattern which it compares with inputs of the person's current position to determine if it is "normal or not." If the person is put into an obviously better posture, it will appear wrong to that person. It then takes time for a new posture to be built up. He also found that when the postural muscles of the back increase in activity to maintain the upright posture then the trunk muscles are freed and respiration improves. He summerizes this research in his work *The Lost Sixth Sense.*

In 1992, Dr. John Austin published his study of the Alexander Technique's influence on breathing. He concluded that it demonstrated "a strong association between a course of Alexander Technique instruction and an increase in measures of respiratory muscular strength and endurance." He also identified four possible mechanisms to account for the changes:

1 Increased length of the muscles of the torso.

2 Increased strength and/or endurance of muscles of the abdominal wall.

3 Decreased resting tensions of chest wall muscles.

4 Enhanced coordination of the respiratory muscles.

Austin saw these changes as indirect results of the lengthening in stature and the "subjects developing particular appreciation of head neck elongation and poise."

BELOW *The control of human and animal movement is improved by the use of the Alexander Technique.*

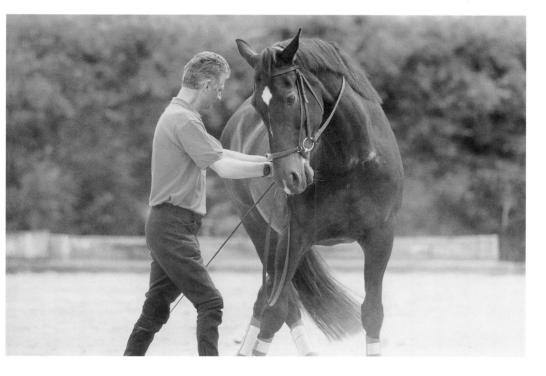

EVOLUTION

Alexander soon became known as the "breathing man" because of his ability to breathe effortlessly and noiselessly when acting or reciting. The importance of the freedom of breathing extends beyond voice use.

Breathing is the process not only of bringing air into the lungs, but also of transporting the oxygen around so it can reach the cells that need it. The Alexander Technique not only brings about deeper and calmer breathing, but because all the muscles are releasing and expanding, it allows the blood – and thereby oxygen – to flow in an uninterrupted way. In this way, breathing becomes easier and the efficient blood-flow ensures sufficient oxygen is supplied.

Alexander criticized the fashion for "deep breathing" exercies. He argued that the idea of taking a deep breath is simply counterproductive. Similarly, chest exercises do not increase air capacity; they simply build muscles on the outside of the ribs, and make the chest look bigger. For an expansion and enlargement of the lungs to happen, the whole body needs to release and expand. This only happens when the whole muscular system is coordinated.

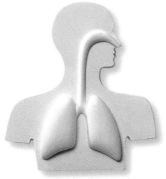

ABOVE *Bad breathing is only a symptom of poor co-ordination. The standard of breathing depends on the standard of use of the psychophysical mechanism.*

When doctors realized that Alexander had discovered something new and remarkable, he was persuaded to introduce his method in London, where he moved in 1904. He soon established a thriving practice, initially teaching members of the theatrical profession, but also people who had been recommended by their doctors to see him. In the early evening he traveled between West End theaters, helping actors to prepare for their performances (among them Henry Irving, Herbert Beerbohm Tree, and Lily Brayton).

In 1909 his Technique was proposed as a physical education system for Australian schools. Dr. A. Leeper, commissioned by the Australian Board of Education, examined methods of physical education in England and concluded in his report that he would "without hesitation" give "the first place to the system associated with the name of Mr. F. Matthias Alexander."

Despite this warm recommendation Dr. Leeper's advice was ignored by the Australian School Board. However, Alexander received much encouragement from many other people. His holistic view of health was supported by Dr. J. E. R. McDonagh in his work *The Nature of Disease* (1931–36). McDonagh agreed that the wrong use of the body played an important role in the nature of disease, suggesting that Alexander's work could be described as the first clinical physiology for the human being.

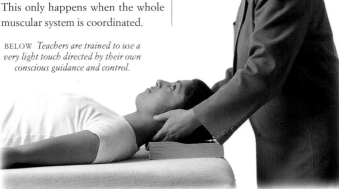

BELOW *Teachers are trained to use a very light touch directed by their own conscious guidance and control.*

When he speaks
The air, a chartered libertine,
is still
And the mute wonder lurketh
in men's ears
To steal his sweet and honeyed
sentences...

**WILLIAM SHAKESPEARE:
HENRY V**

ALEXANDER'S WRITINGS

1910 Man's Supreme Inheritance

In 1910 Alexander published *Man's Supreme Inheritance* in which he proposed an evolutionary explanation for the general deterioration in health and well-being of modern man. The course of evolution had allowed adaptation to be a gradual one. Man's present state reflected his inability to adapt himself to the rapidly changing circumstances of civilized life. Reliance on subconscious guidance of the mental and bodily processes was no longer successful. Our "supreme inheritance" was the possibility of passing from subconscious to conscious control of ourselves. He argued against the unconscious pursuit of exercise, relaxation, and deep-breathing methods as remedies because they did not deal with the underlying cause of misuse, which was unreliable sensory appreciation. Conscious control involved:
a) an ability to inhibit habitual interference with the upright posture;
b) an ability freely to control the motivating factors responsible for misusing the body, as well as an ability to consciously direct the body into an efficient posture and working state;
c) an ability to maintain improved functioning in all activities, especially when facing unfamiliar circumstances. Because of the unity of mind and body, a habit could never be thought of as simply mental or physical, but recognized as a unified response of the whole self. A habit involved a deterioration of the muscular sense that makes it difficult to distinguish between appropriate and inappropriate effort, a need for the habit, and mental resistance or laziness. Changing habits required a recognition of true body poise, together with an understanding of the inhibitory and volitional powers of the mind.

1924 Constructive Conscious Control

In this second book, Alexander discussed sensory appreciation in its relation to evolutionary development, and human beings' needs and happiness.

Our ancestors had displayed good body use, which was controlled by instinct. However, these instincts did not equip them for the rapid advances and changing circumstances of modern civilized life. He argued that, on the whole, we lacked the grace and poise of our ancestors. Restoration of sensory appreciation to a reliable standard was essential.

Alexander introduced the term "end-gaining." It was used to describe directly proceeding to gain a desired end which resulted in an unsatisfactory use of ourselves. Alexander suggested adopting the principle that he termed "the means whereby." This involved a willingness to pay attention to the process with which an end is achieved, resulting in a more satisfactory use of ourselves.

He argued that our conception of an idea or an instruction depends on our standard of sensory appreciation. Most teaching is based on the incorrect assumption that having asked someone to do something, they will be able to do it. He exposed the fallacy of correcting a defect when sensory appreciation was unreliable and advised the re-education of the whole person. A recognition of this unreliable sensory appreciation was the first step to correcting a defect.

During the process of learning the Alexander Technique, pupils began to stop end-gaining and trying to be right. He argued that the inability to attend to two things at once is an indication of poor sensory awareness often resulting in stress and misdirected effort.

1931 The Use of the Self

In this book Alexander made some important observations concerning human behavior. Instinctive misdirection was associated with the untrustworthiness of feeling and an instinctive response to stimuli. He reasoned that feeling could be made trustworthy again.

Alexander discussed how our reflex functioning and our reactions to stimuli were conditioned by the use of the whole self. The direction of the body, which is monitored and organized by instinct, has become more and more a misdirection, resulting in symptoms of mental disorder, disease, and poor reflex functioning. By teaching the technique of conscious redirection of the stature, general functioning could be indirectly improved.

His technique did not involve dealing with specific symptoms directly, but established a general direction of use which was the basis for improved psychophysical functioning.

1941 The Universal Constant in Living

Alexander argued that we can coordinate and control muscle use to our best advantage. He stated that the performance of physical exercises, while still under the influence of unreliable sensory appreciation, uses the very sensory processes that need correction, and could therefore not be beneficial and may even tend to aggravate the problem.

Alexander encouraged his pupils to inhibit their response to any stimulus. Simple activities, such as sitting down in a chair or getting up from a chair, allowed pupils to have a new sensory experience of a more upright stature with the accompanying sense of increased freedom in movement.

THE SOCIETY

A few years before F. M. Alexander's death, discussions began about the formation of a professional society to supervise standards of teaching and teacher training, and in 1958 the Society of Teachers of the Alexander Technique (S.T.A.T.) was formed in Britain with the following aims:

BELOW John Nicholls, Director of the Brighton Alexander Training Center, instructs his student in the refined use of her hands and directed use of herself.

1 To maintain and improve professional standards.
2 To make the Technique more widely known.
3 To facilitate contact between members.
4 To encourage research.
5 To prevent abuse and exploitation by untrained people.

At that time, in 1958, three Alexander teacher training courses had been running in Britain. By 2001 there were 14 approved by S.T.A.T. in the UK, and courses in at least nine other countries approved either by S.T.A.T. or by similar professional societies set up more recently in those countries. The Society assesses the suitability of

those who wish to run teacher raining courses and lays down minimum requirements in terms of length of training, structure of training, and core curriculum. There is also a system of visits by external moderators to try to maintain equivalence of qualification standards among courses. Because the nature of the work is so individual, courses are small, ranging from 5 to 40 trainees, and a teacher–student ratio of about 1:5 is recommended. Classes usually take place for 3–4 hours a day, four or, more commonly, five days a week, still following the basic pattern established by Alexander himself, as that level of consistency and continuity has been found to be most beneficial.

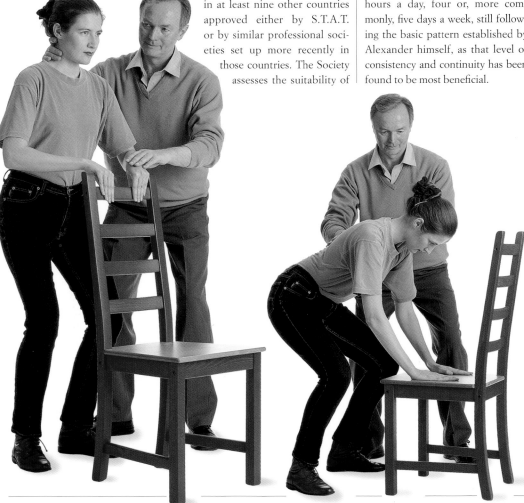

TRAINING COURSES – JOHN NICHOLLS

Students on John Nicholls' teacher training course tell this joke: Student arrives home looking weary after morning on the training course. Partner asks sympathetically: "You look worn out. What did you do in class today?" Student replies: "Oh, I lay on the floor for a while, then I went in and out of a chair a few times, walked a few steps, lay down again, sat with my hands on the back of another chair, and then put my hands on someone else while they stood up and sat down. I am absolutely exhausted!"

Indeed, an Alexander teacher-training class does look like a group of people repeatedly performing mundane, simple activities with great care and attention. Yet the tiredness is real, especially during the first year of the training, as these simple procedures put demands on muscles to work in new ways, and the clarity of attention required is almost like building up new "mental" muscle.

Alexander's first attempts at training others to teach his work were of an informal apprenticeship nature. His brother A. R. and his sister Amy had assisted him in Melbourne, and in London he took on Ethel Webb and Irene Tasker as assistants in a similar fashion. However, in 1931 a more organized training program began. From the beginning it was a three-year program, with students meeting for several hours, five days a week, during the typical British educational term times. The emphasis was largely on students working to

BELOW *The attention required to re-educate the body develops a kind of "mental muscle".*

Make it your ambition to lead a quiet life, to mind your own business, and to work with your hands.

I THESSALONIANS 4: 11

develop their own use of the Technique to a very high level, as Alexander firmly believed from his own experience of teaching that you must practice what you preach.

In the work of kinesthetic (or sensory) re-education, the good use of the teacher is paramount in determining whether his hands succeed in conveying to the pupil the sensory experience of the coordination required, and only personal experience can enable a teacher to give the clear verbal explanations that are also necessary.

After Alexander's death in 1955, the course was carried on by Walter Carrington.

RIGHT *Theory and practice always go together in the Alexander Technique training.*

Walter and his wife Dilys Carrington have maintained this link with Alexander, and added extra structural elements to the training, such as regular study of Alexander's books and other relevant literature, study of anatomy and physiology, and a more organized approach to the development of the manual skills of Alexander teaching. The majority of training courses today proceed along these lines.

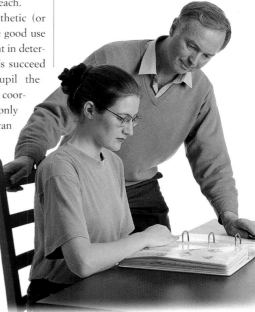

LEARNING FOR LIFE

When someone is having individual lessons in the Alexander Technique, a process of change and improvement takes place by frequent repetition of simple activities under the guidance of the teacher. Emphasis is on the quality of attention to the pupil's use of the Technique as the activity is performed, so the ends to be gained may seem relatively easy, but the quality of performance is all-important, rather than success. An analogous process takes place in the training of Alexander teachers. The actual maneuvers a teacher performs with hands on a pupil really look quite simple: moving someone in and out of a chair; gently holding and guiding their head, neck, torso, and limbs in sitting, standing, and while the pupil lies on a firm couch. Can this really take three years to learn, especially when compared to the apparently complex manual skills of, say, osteopathy or chiropractic? But as with the individual lesson process, the secret lies in the quality of performance: learning to

do simple things with a very high degree of coordinated use; the teacher's whole body expressing the light, lively, integrated, elastic muscle tone he or she is aiming to convey to the pupil. This is not just a matter of being a good visual role model. We have found from many years' experience that the "tone" of

the experience conveyed by the teacher's hands is a reflection of the tone of the teacher's entire body. The external simplicity hides a skill that will go on being refined throughout the teacher's working life.

A teacher therefore has to learn to achieve this coordinated expansion with hands on a pupil, and to maintain it while doing any further necessary muscular work, moving a pupil's head, arm, or leg, for example. Thus any muscular activity required on the part of the teacher is spread throughout his whole body, not producing a build-up of shortened, tense muscle in any one part. This way of working constantly conveys a releasing, integrating, expansive stimulus to the pupil, both at rest and in movement.

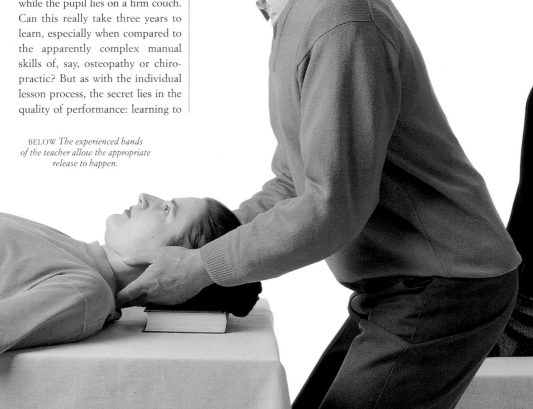

BELOW *The experienced hands of the teacher allow the appropriate release to happen.*

USE OF HANDS

Alexander Technique teachers give precise verbal instructions reinforced by use of their hands. In most forms of what might be termed "manual therapy," for example, physiotherapy or osteopathy, there are two distinct modes of using the hands. They are used to feel, to palpate and discover what the problems are in the patient; then they are used to intervene, to perform some type of manipulative maneuver in order to correct the perceived problem.

A distinct feature of good Alexander teaching is that these two modes are unified: that use of the teacher's whole self that makes for greatest sensitivity in the hands to feel what is happening in the pupil is at the same time the key aspect of conveying to the pupil the possibility of change to a better manner of use.

One of Alexander's most useful discoveries was the practical procedure known as "Hands on the back of the chair." It provides a paradigm for all use of the hands in activity, ensuring that the use of the hands is coordinated with the primary needs of the trunk for upright support and freedom to breathe. Alexander himself is often quoted by teachers who trained with him as saying this procedure contained all the experiences one needed to use the hands as a teacher of the Technique. The "hands on the back of the chair procedure" therefore provides the background to all the learning required to use one's hands on others in an Alexander teaching program. This learning is best done in small groups, being guided through a step-by-step program over the first two years of the

course. In this way, simple practices become the basis from which more complex skills can develop. It is a steady, well-worked-out discipline, which needs to be established before students become able to work more fluidly as they near the end of their period of training.

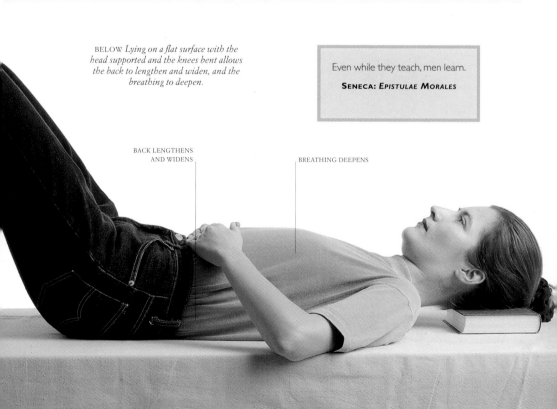

BELOW *Lying on a flat surface with the head supported and the knees bent allows the back to lengthen and widen, and the breathing to deepen.*

Even while they teach, men learn.

SENECA: *EPISTULAE MORALES*

BACK LENGTHENS
AND WIDENS

BREATHING DEEPENS

The Use of the Self

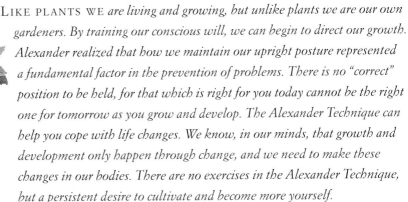

LIKE PLANTS WE *are living and growing, but unlike plants we are our own gardeners. By training our conscious will, we can begin to direct our growth. Alexander realized that how we maintain our upright posture represented a fundamental factor in the prevention of problems. There is no "correct" position to be held, for that which is right for you today cannot be the right one for tomorrow as you grow and develop. The Alexander Technique can help you cope with life changes. We know, in our minds, that growth and development only happen through change, and we need to make these changes in our bodies. There are no exercises in the Alexander Technique, but a persistent desire to cultivate and become more yourself.*

ABOVE *Like plants, we change as we grow and develop. The Alexander Technique helps us to cope with these changes.*

USE AFFECTS FUNCTIONING

We use most things for a limited amount of time, then stop to go on to do something else. However, unlike tools and instruments our minds and bodies are in constant use. Most of the time we are not aware of this. As you use a kitchen knife, you are conscious of the knife and what you are cutting. Does it need sharpening? Is the handle getting a bit loose? Is it clean? Is it too near your fingers? You will be aware of the implement and its state. If it is not working well enough, you immediately try and fix it. Have you ever thought that you might need fixing? How are you holding the knife? Perhaps you are grip-

Our bodies are gardens to the which our wills are gardeners so that if we plant nettles or sow lettuce, set hyssop and weed up thyme, supply it with one gender of herbs or distract it with many, either to have it sterile with idleness or manured with industry.

WILLIAM SHAKESPEARE:
OTHELLO

ping it too tightly, holding your breath as you chop, clenching your jaw, tensing your shoulders, bracing your knees? These reactions may affect your level of skill and efficiency or wear you out.

If we use ourselves in a better way, we function more efficiently. Tension in the back muscles will shorten the spine, which normally bends the spine forward. There is a very simple experiment that you

can try that makes it easy to see how the way you use something can increase or decrease its length. If you take a stick of a certain length and bend it, you will shorten the distance between both ends. If you bend yourself in such a way, you will shorten yourself by shortening and contracting your muscles. How your muscles operate affects your functioning. If you pull down, you will be restricting internal organs, stiffening your joints, limiting your breathing. All these may lead to problems and loss of vitality and enjoyment.

When you begin to pay attention to yourself, you can change how you use your mind and body, then your posture and physiology will change. The functioning of the circulatory system is changed, and as a consequence blood pressure is stabilized. Over the years by doing things habitually we have become less conscious. We do not think about how we use ourselves. To change we have to recognise habits limit us.

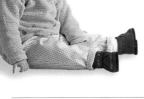

LEFT *Young children display natural good use of the body as they have not formed any bad habits.*

SHORT VERSUS TALL

TALL

Tall
When you are neither collapsed nor trying to stand up too straight, your muscles and bones have a chance to achieve their full potential length. Compare gently holding a stick at both ends; the distance between both ends is not shortened.

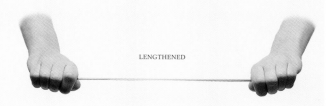

LENGTHENED

SHORT

Short
When the body is collapsed down in front and the head pulled down, the bones and muscles cannot lengthen, and you shorten. Compare bending the stick, when the distance between the two ends becomes shortened.

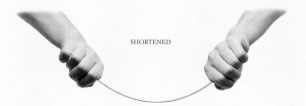

SHORTENED

SHORT

Short
When you pull your back in and push up your chest to try to stand up straight, you actually make yourself shorter. Compare bending the stick the opposite way; the distance between the ends is still shortened.

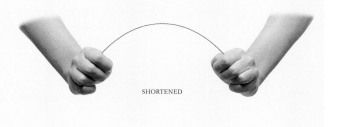

SHORTENED

Of habits devil, is angel yet in this,
That aptly is put on. Refrain
to-night;
And that shall lend a kind
of easiness
To the next abstinence; the next
more easy;
For use almost can change the
stamp of nature…

WILLIAM SHAKESPEARE:
HAMLET

HABITS

Habits are formed by repeating actions until they become settled, regular activities that are often hard to give up. When we first learn to do something, whether it is a basic skill like walking or a more refined, complicated skill like playing an instrument or handling a tennis racket, we need to think about what we are doing. As we practice the skill, we still have to be conscious of what we are doing, but eventually it becomes automatic, a habit.

We may turn left on a journey because that is what we always do, although today we needed to turn right. In this way we become slaves to our habits, and it becomes more difficult to be open to changes in our lives. Then change becomes something difficult we have to do, instead of being exciting and inviting. In order to change a habit we have to go back to the time when we originally learned the skill. We have to change our response from being unconscious of what we are doing to being more aware and conscious. We need to think about what we are doing. Have you ever gone to lift an empty box which you expected to be heavy? Often we generate far more effort than we need, and this imposes too much muscular tension on the body. It can become a vicious circle. Each time we use a certain amount of effort in an activity, like speaking, we will use it again because the effort becomes so closely associated with the act of speaking. When a habit is ingrained,

it will feel as if we cannot speak unless we produce this effort. We need to have a way we can put this change into effect. The principles needed to break habits are conscious inhibition and conscious direction. We must ask ourselves first what do we want. In order to avoid habitual reactions, we need to stop briefly before proceeding.

BREAKING HABITS

If an attempt is to be made to change a person's habit, two things are essential. The first is an adequate desire, on the part of the subject, to make the change. The helper needs to use his ingenuity to build up a degree of motivation in the subject. In addition, the person with the habit has to be brought to a condition in which he is aware of the "feel" of this changing condition which will, if allowed to proceed, lead to the habitual movement. Once this moment is recognized, he can interpose an alternative behavior pattern.

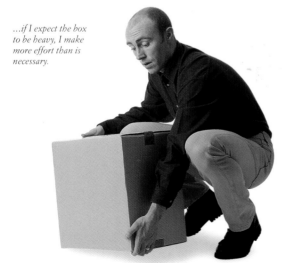

…if I expect the box to be heavy, I make more effort than is necessary.

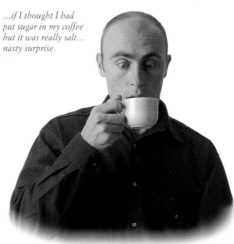

…if I thought I had put sugar in my coffee but it was really salt… nasty surprise.

CONSCIOUS INHIBITION

Inhibition is the practice of pausing before an action. It gives us the time that is needed to register "how" we are preparing for any activity and whether excessive muscular tension is present. The inhibitory process enables a release of the unnecessary contraction so that the lengthening and widening of the body musculature can be restored. Inhibition is a positive process, leading to release, efficient preparation, and optimum readiness. Why don't we think before we act? In *The Use of the Self*, Alexander said:

...I came to see at last that if I was ever to be able to change my habitual use and dominate my instinctive direction, it would be necessary for me to make the experience of receiving the stimulus to speak and refusing to do anything immediately in response.

By stopping our habitual reactions, we give ourselves a chance to prevent mistakes and to give ourselves time to make a choice about how we proceed. As our mental attitude changes, there is a chance to break our habits. Frank Pierce Jones said in *Freedom to Change*:

Inhibition is a positive, not a negative force. Some degree of inhibition is essential not only for a good life but for any life at all... Inhibition is a physiological process which does not need to be conscious in order to operate. Bringing it up to the conscious level not only establishes an indirect control over anti-gravity responses but facilitates the learning of new habits and the unlearning of those that are old and unwanted. When a stimulus is presented for the

BELOW *Pausing to think before taking an action enables us to assess unnecessary muscular tension.*

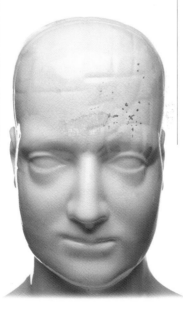

first time, many responses are available, including not making a response at all. If one of these responses is selected and learned, it can be repeated without loss of choice as long as the process remains conscious. If it drops below the level of consciousness, a "set" will be established linking the stimulus with the response, which will then occur automatically whether it is appropriate or not... The result is a habit which operates unconsciously (like an innate reflex) and which is resistant to change. Inhibition raises the level of tonic activity in the nervous system, brings the operation of the habit to a conscious level, and restores choice (including the choice of making the original response).

CONSCIOUS DIRECTION

All the time in life, we are giving ourselves directions. We have conversations with ourselves about what we want to happen. "Smarten up, pull yourself together, get real, try hard, don't give up, get your act together, don't go wrong." We can give ourselves these instructions to find our way, as we follow directions on a map. As we map-read, we work out where we are and in which direction we need to go. Always we are going from here to there. When we are lost, we are grateful for any information that is clearly and confidently given – we need direction; our language is full of references to "being led," "following our guiding star," "taking the right path," "being out of line," "on the wrong track." We often know when we are off course. Alexander

HEAD GOES
FORWARD AND UP

NECK IS FREE

BACK
LENGTHENS
AND WIDENS

LEFT *Conscious directions enable the body to release, lengthen and widen, restoring the shape that nature intended.*

> JACK: "You're quite perfect, Miss Fairfax."
> GWENDOLEN: "Oh! I hope I am not that. It would leave no room for developments, and I intend to develop in many directions."
>
> **OSCAR WILDE:**
> *THE IMPORTANCE OF BEING EARNEST*

observed that certain directions are not as helpful as others. We cannot see directions, but we can see the result of them in the posture and form of ourselves. Alexander formulated the directions "Let the neck be free so that the head can go forward and up and so that the back can lengthen and widen" to give himself a clear route to follow.

Conscious directions are instructions given to enable the body to release, lengthen, and widen. It is by giving conscious directions that we encourage our bodies to adopt their full stature. Direction does not involve a direct command; rather it is a process of giving suggestions that encourage a reflex process to happen and avoid interference with the natural poise of our upright posture.

There exists in these directions an implicit message that we have to give ourselves time for this to happen. These directions

can enable us to come back to the shape that nature intended. If we have no directions, or choose not to follow them, then we could get lost.

END-GAINING AND MEANS-WHEREBY

In the 1930s Aldous Huxley had lessons from Alexander from which he benefited tremendously. He believed that the Alexander Technique was unique in its ability to deal with the problem of "end-gaining." "End-gaining" describes the process in which a person is preoccupied with goals and disregards how the "means-whereby" the goals are attained. At worst, "end-gaining" advocates the end at any cost, an obsession with outcomes with no regard to the cost to the psycho-physical organism. Huxley (quoted in Frank Pierce Jones, *Freedom to Change*) said:

> One has to make the discovery for oneself, starting from scratch and to find what old F.M. Alexander called "the means-whereby," without which good intentions merely pave hell, and the idealist remains an ineffectual, self-destructive and other-destructive end-gainer.

The Alexander Technique encourages you to observe and think about how you work to gain your end. The basic learning skills that any child develops rely on this way of learning. The child is told to think about what he is doing, to take his time, to take care, and not to rush. These instructions are the "means-whereby" the child gains his ends. When not enough attention is paid to how that end is gained, problems can arise. Have you ever found that the harder you try, the more difficult it is to achieve what you want? Let me give you an example:

If you perform breathing exercises in order to have a greater lung capacity, you could be actually creating more tensions in your body and undermining your inherent potential to breathe naturally, fully, and freely. Because you are concentrating on the exercise of breathing and trying too hard to achieve results too quickly, you will be defeating yourself. When you "end-gain," you can block results because you generate excessive muscular tension throughout your body in your determination to get what you want.

Often it seems to us that our day consists of a long list of activities, things we have to get done. We rush through these tasks as quickly as possible to get to the time when we can relax. We end up not enjoying our daily activities because they have become unpleasant tasks. Sometimes they have become painful activities because of the excessive muscular tension we have created as we rush to try to get them over and done with. It is a vicious circle that can be broken by attending to the means whereby we gain

RIGHT *Children's basic learning skills are the "means-whereby" they achieve their goal. Alexander encouraged us to pay attention to this process.*

our ends. The Technique enables us to develop the sensitivity that gives us a more accurate perception of ourselves and how act. We strive to be "on time," and tend to forget that we also need to be "in time."

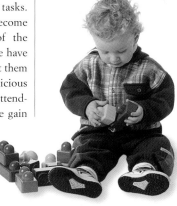

DIRECTION

As an animal walks forward, the head is in a direct horizontal line with the spine. The movement of the head goes in the same direction as the movement of the body. The head acts as a balancer, regulating the weight carried by the front and hind legs as it is lowered or raised, usually toward food. In the two legged animal, man, the head has to move forward while the spine is in a vertical direction. The demands of these different directions creates the need for a unique balancing act.

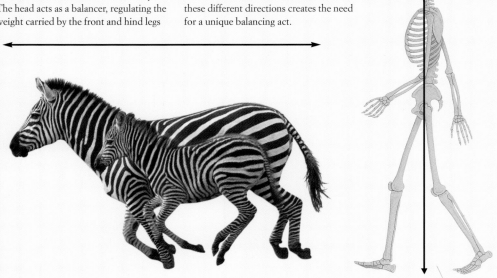

SENSORY APPRECIATION: THE SEARCHLIGHT OF ATTENTION

We are familiar with our five senses: taste, touch, sight, smell, hearing. Sensory appreciation is our conscious evaluation of these senses. Perhaps you have never realized that you have a sixth sense, proprioception. This is the ability to understand and use the signals that your balance mechanism and movement receptors send to your brain.

A lot of the time we are unaware that we have this sixth sense, yet we do not feel quite right. Like Hamlet we feel, "like sweet bells, jangled and out of tune." This is because we are unaware of ourselves. Have you ever looked at a photograph of yourself and been surprised by what you see – "I don't look like that! I didn't realize I was doing that!" Have you caught a reflection of yourself in a window and been surprised at how you are standing.

When you look in a mirror, you can see what you are doing. This can cause quite a shock – back hollowed, head pulled back, knees locked. As you change to a "better" posture, the new one can look and feel wrong to you. You are used to your old body position, so the new posture pattern seems strange. It takes time to adopt a new posture, even though the benefits are obvious both visually and in your physiological functioning and general well-

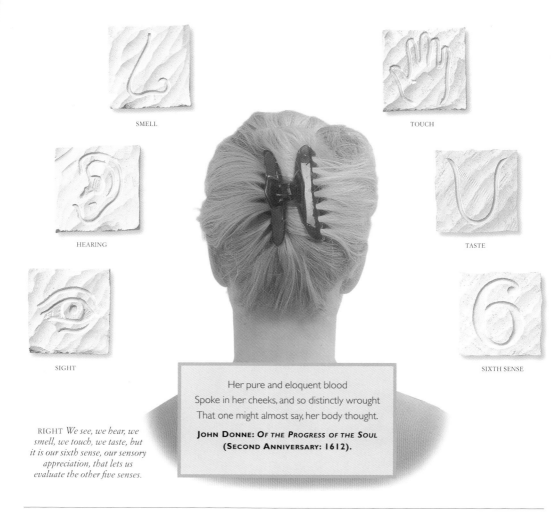

SMELL

TOUCH

HEARING

TASTE

SIGHT

SIXTH SENSE

Her pure and eloquent blood
Spoke in her cheeks, and so distinctly wrought
That one might almost say, her body thought.

**JOHN DONNE: *OF THE PROGRESS OF THE SOUL*
(SECOND ANNIVERSARY: 1612).**

RIGHT *We see, we hear, we smell, we touch, we taste, but it is our sixth sense, our sensory appreciation, that lets us evaluate the other five senses.*

being. Dr. G.E. Coghill, in the *Appreciation for The Universal Constant in Living*, said:

> Alexander has further demonstrated the very important psychological principle that the proprioceptive system can be brought under conscious control and can be educated to carry to the motor centers the stimulus that is responsible for the muscular activity that brings about the manner of working (use) of the mechanism of correct posture.

THE ALEXANDER TECHNIQUE BRINGS YOU TO YOUR SENSES

Alexander showed that it is possible to be unaware of what we are doing. It is generally assumed that feelings give us accurate information about our bodies. When this feedback is incorrect, our sensory appreciation becomes unreliable. In connection with unreliable sensory appreciation the following story was related by Alexander in his book *Constructive Conscious Control*:

> A little girl who had been unable to walk properly for some years was brought to the writer for a diagnosis of the defects in the use of the psychophysical mechanisms that were responsible for her more or less crippled state. When this had been done, a request was made that a demonstration should be given to those present of the manipulative side of the work so that certain readjustments and coordinations might be temporally secured, thus showing, in keeping with the diagnosis, the possibilities of re-education on a general basis in a

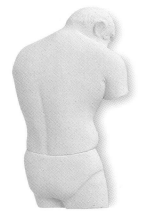

ABOVE *It is all too easy to be unaware of your habitual stance and posture. A close examination in the mirror may reveal surprising bad habits.*

> case of this kind. The demonstration was successful from this point of view. For the time being, the child's body was comparatively straightened out – that is, without the extreme twists and distortions that had been so noticeable when she came into the room. When this was done, the little girl looked across at her mother and said to her in an indescribable tone, "Oh, Mommy, he has pulled me all out of shape." Her deceptive feelings led this little girl to believe that she was standing straight, when she was all out of shape. We are often under the same misconception. What we do feels right because it is our habitual way of acting, no matter how wrong and unsatisfactory it is in reality.

Change involves carrying out an activity that goes against the habits of a lifetime. This is certainly one of the most challenging aspects of practicing the Alexander Technique, but the reward is a more finely-tuned sense of ourselves.

PROPRIOCEPTION

Proprioception is a term first used by the eminent neurophysiologist Sir Charles Sherrington. It is our secret sixth sense. It is the process through which human beings get information from their bodies, ascertain their position in space, and recognize whether too much muscular effort is being used. This instinctive and unconscious process has developed and acted as a trustworthy guide throughout the course of evolution, ensuring correct and efficient posture and ease in movement. Sensory appreciation allows us to consciously receive and evaluate this information and lets us know whether our body is functioning well. Refined sensory appreciation improves the feedback from all the senses.

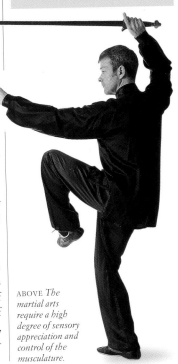

ABOVE *The martial arts require a high degree of sensory appreciation and control of the musculature.*

27

PRIMARY CONTROL

Everybody who has a head, neck, and back has a primary control, the processes that control the use of the head and neck in relation to the back. It is primary because it comes first in every movement. To a large extent it determines the coordination and muscle tones of the rest of the body. The parts of the body should be used in harmony with the primary control, that coordinated action of the head, neck, and back working together, creating a total pattern of use. Alexander discovered, through carefully observing his movements in the mirror, that he habitually interfered with his head-neck-back relationship.

That the neck is of great importance for the control of balance and posture in animals has been known since the 19th century, when vivisectionists showed that cutting the posterior neck muscles resulted in severe disturbances of posture and locomotion in animals.

When the head is forward and up, the weight of the body is back, the spine lengthened, a balanced, upright posture results. When the head is back and down, the body weight forward, and the spine shortened, a stooped posture is created. The delicate balance of the head on the neck can be upset quite easily. Sensory input from the neck muscles is very important physiologically. The number of nerve receptors in neck muscles is much higher than in other muscles. The control of muscles in posture and movement is primarily affected by the state of neck muscles with their very strong sensory input to the brain.

The procedures used in the Alexander Technique help establish a new dynamic balance among the forces acting on the head, so that more of the postural work can be done by disks, and ligaments and muscles acting at their optimal length. The head feels lighter because more of its weight is carried by lengthened muscles. The increase in the axis of head rotation facilitates extension of the spine. The space between all the vertebrae, particularly between the first vertebra and the head increases, creating more room for blood vessels so that more blood flows to the brain.

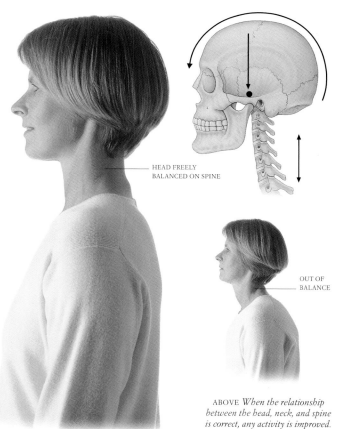

HEAD FREELY
BALANCED ON SPINE

OUT OF
BALANCE

ABOVE *When the relationship between the head, neck, and spine is correct, any activity is improved.*

Anatomy: The Structure

WHAT DETERMINES OUR SHAPE? *Growth patterns, genetic endowment,*
environment, education, training, life experiences, trauma, success, potential – tapped,
untapped. We are changing position all the time, so our shape is constantly changing.
Shape is roughly determined by bones and muscles. Bone is a living substance, capable
of great changes, including degeneration. Muscles can adopt very different shapes
and maintain them through constant use and misuse.

All muscles in animals, including humans, are in a state of mild contraction even when seemingly still. Maintaining a static (unmoving) posture demands muscular activity just as any movement does. Just to stand, the muscles that oppose one another on either side of the knee, hip, and ankle must exert an equal and opposite tension. This stabilizes the joints and prevents them from collapsing under the body's weight. Movement is simply the change from one stance to the next. When you move one of your limbs, you increase the state of contraction on one side of the joint and decrease a proportional amount on the other side. When a "good" posture is adopted, it means that the contractions of the muscles are adequate to maintain the body in such a way that favors the best functioning and puts minimal strain on the muscles, tendons, ligaments, and bones. The reverse is true of the effects of "bad" posture. Besides the obvious detraction from appearance, poor posture makes you tire more quickly. Abnormal pulls are put on tendons, ligaments, joints, and bones, and can lead to deformities. Poor posture

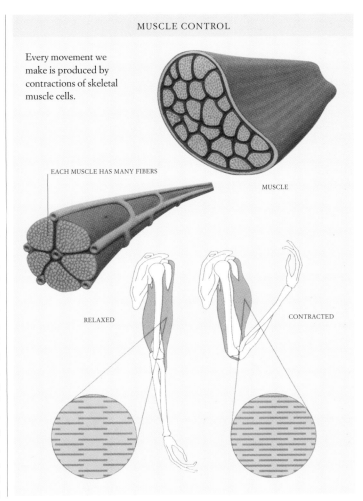

MUSCLE CONTROL

Every movement we make is produced by contractions of skeletal muscle cells.

EACH MUSCLE HAS MANY FIBERS

MUSCLE

RELAXED

CONTRACTED

decreases the breathing capacity of the lungs. Posture directly affects your bodily functions. We often associate good posture with being straight, and poor posture with being bent. However, there is nothing straight in the human body. Everything is designed on the principle of curves. These curves are developed as a baby learns to hold up its head and stand, and provide balance in the upright position (refer to the section "Growth and Development of the Child," pages 74–75). They give strength to support the weight of the rest of the body. A curved structure has more strength than a straight one made of the same material of the same size.

The dictionary defines man as "an individual of the highest type of animal existing, especially in his extraordinary mental development." The Latin name for man is *Homo sapiens* – translated as the "thinking man."

THE AXIAL SKELETON

The bones of the skull, spine, and chest, and the hyoid bone in the neck, make up the axial skeleton.

The Skull

The skull is made up of 28 bones. Eight of these form the cranium, 14 form the face, and six form the middle ear. These bones protect the brain and also carry and protect the important sense organs of the eyes, ears, and nose. The skull is not solid bone, which would be impossibly heavy, but has sinuses, which are spaces inside the cranium. The bone at the base of the skull (occiput) makes a joint with the top vertebra

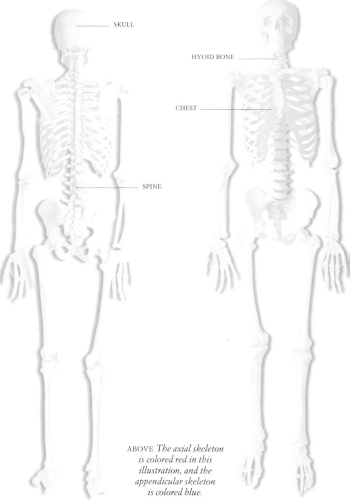

SKULL

HYOID BONE

CHEST

SPINE

ABOVE *The axial skeleton is colored red in this illustration, and the appendicular skeleton is colored blue.*

of the spinal column which allows the head to pivot on the first (atlas) vertebra and rotate on the second (axis) vertebra. This joint (atlanto occipital) enables the skull to nod and turn, crucial to the freedom of our upright posture and our entire movement pattern. The spinal cord enters the cranium through a large hole (foranum magnum) in the occipital bone. The upper jaw (maxilla) is part of the skull, but the

lower jaw is hinged for movement by a condyloid joint that permits all types of movement except rotation, including opening, closing, sliding, chewing, crushing.

The Vertebrae (Spinal Column)

The spinal column needs to meet two contradictory mechanical requirements – stability and mobility. It consists of 24 individual vertebrae made up of bone, with a channel in the middle through which the spinal cord, a bundle of nerve pathways running from the brain, passes. In this position the cord is protected from damage. Each vertebra is separated from the next one by an intervertebral disk made of fibrous cartilage that acts as a shock-absorbing cushion. These disks conform to the size of the vertebrae. They not only absorb any shock that may be delivered to the spinal column, but also aid in its mobility.

The Breastbone and Ribs

The breastbone (sternum) is shaped like a dagger, with the bone ending with a piece of cartilage called the xiphoid process. It forms the point of articulation for the collarbone (clavicle) and is the anterior attachment point for the ribs. The ribs 1–10 are anchored to the 12 thoracic vertebrae, but ribs 11 and 12, floating ribs, are not attached to the front. The bone of the rib is called the shaft and is somewhat flattened. The lower border of the shaft has a costal groove that protects the blood

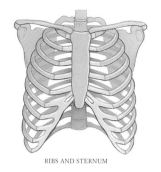

RIBS AND STERNUM

vessels and nerves that course along each rib.

These 12 pairs of ribs form a bony cage known as the chest (or thorax). The ribcage is shaped like a barrel with ribs 1–7 getting larger, then 7–12 getting progressively smaller. The lungs lie enclosed within an airtight thoracic cavity. The structure of the chest cavity is such that its volume can be made to increase or decrease. The skeletal framework is almost completely filled with lungs and heart. The dimensions of the thoracic cavity can increase in three planes during inhalation – the top, around the sides, and down to the diaphragm.

BELOW *The spinal vertebrae and disks work together to ensure that the spinal column is both mobile, and adequately protected.*

TRANSVERSE PROCESS

TRANSVERSE PROCESS

BODY

SPINAL CANAL

BODY

THE APPENDICULAR SKELETON

The limbs are movable appendages. There are 126 bones in the appendicular skeleton, which consists of the bones of the upper and lower extremities, and of the pectoral girdle and the pelvic girdle.

Bones of the Upper Extremities

The shoulder girdle (pectoral girdle) includes the clavicle and scapula (shoulder blade) and with the arms, wrists, and hands, comprises the bones of the upper extremities. The clavicle is essentially a strut that projects the scapula far enough laterally to clear the barrel-shaped chest wall. The scapula carries the arm and is a thin, flat, triangular plate of bone covered with muscles on both sides. It lies freely movable on the posterior–superior wall of the ribcage.

RIGHT *The upper appendicular skeleton comprises a total of 126 bones.*

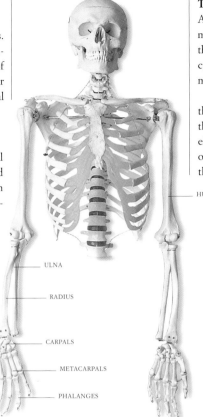

ULNA

RADIUS

CARPALS

METACARPALS

PHALANGES

HUMERUS

The Arm

Attached to the scapula at its proximal end is the long upper bone of the arm (humerus). Long bones are cylinders of hard bone with soft marrow on the inside.

The upper arm articulates with the two bones (radius and ulna) of the lower arm (forearm) at the elbow joint. The radius is the bone on the thumb side of the lower arm, the ulna is the bone on the little

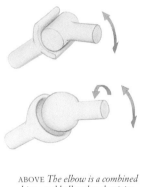

ABOVE *The elbow is a combined hinge and ball-and-socket joint, allowing rotational as well as lateral movement.*

HAND AND WRIST

The wrists and hands have more bones for their size than any other part of the body, 27 bones in all. The tips of the fingers can touch any point in the three-dimensional sphere. The hand is capable of highly complex movements. It gives us the possibility to grip things and carry out delicate, complicated movements that require a high degree of coordination, for example, writing. (See the section "Handwriting," page 54.) The dexterity of our hand movements is one of the distinguishing features of human evolution. Prehension is the essential function of the hand. The thumb can come into contact with each finger. This special movement is called opposition. The hand also gives feedback about thickness and distance to and from the brain, allowing for the development of visual acuity and appreciation.

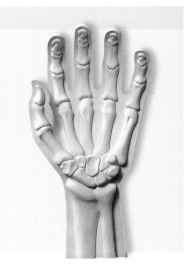

finger side of the lower arm. The elbow is a combined joint. A hinged joint connects the humerus and ulna, and a ball-and-socket joint connects the ulna to the radius, surrounded by synovial membrane, a thin sheet of tissue that allows for freer movement with less friction. This combined joint allows the arm to bend at the elbow and turns the palm upward and downward.

Bones of the Lower Extremities

Two hip bones and the sacrum link to form the pelvic girdle. The long bone of the thigh (femur) forms a deep ball-and-socket joint with the hip bone. The femur articulates with the shin bone (tibia) to form the knee joint. The knee is the intermediate joint of the lower limb. It needs to have great stability and mobility. It is beautifully designed for these two things, but is liable to strains and dislocations. A long slender bone (fibula) lies alongside the tibia, and together they form the top of the ankle joint.

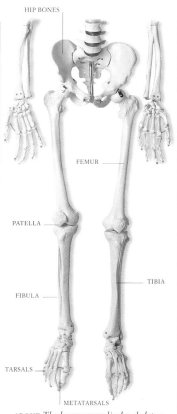

HIP BONES

FEMUR

PATELLA

TIBIA

FIBULA

TARSALS

METATARSALS

ABOVE *The lower appendicular skeleton consists of the bones of the hips, pelvic girdle, legs, ankles, and feet.*

JOINTS

Joints are classified anatomically into two types, mobile or synovial joints, and fixed or fibrous joints. Synovial joints are designed to allow a large range of movements and are lined with a slippery coating called synovium. Fibrous joint movement is stabilizing and is limited by fibrous tissue.

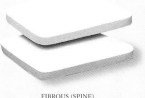

SYNOVIAL (HINGE)

FIBROUS (SPINE)

THE FOOT

There are seven tarsal bones in each foot, which form the heel, back of the foot, and the bottom of the ankle joint, and articulate with five metatarsals, which form the midfoot to which the toes are attached. There are 14 toe bones (phalanges), three in each of the smaller toes and two in each big toe.

The foot needs to be able to support the body's weight, so the bony design forms an arched structure that is reinforced with strong ligaments, allowing for shock absorption and spring in locomotion. Strong ligaments and leg muscle tendons hold the foot bones firmly in position. If the foot tendons or ligaments weaken, the arches flatten and fallen arches or flat feet result. When this malformation happens the spine suffers shocks and the spring reflex of the foot is lost resulting in decreased mobility.

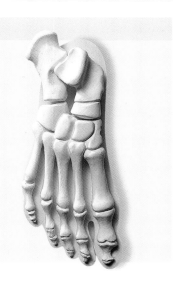

HOW DOES IT ALL LINK UP?

Every bone in the body (with the exception of the hyoid bone) connects to at least one other bone by a joint, making movement possible.

Skeletal Muscle

Skeletal muscle is responsible for body movements, maintaining our upright posture, and generating body heat. Skeletal muscles' main function is to connect bone to bone over a movable joint. The sustained constriction of skeletal muscle can distort natural posture and interfere with the ability to lengthen and widen in stature. Skeletal muscle is activated by messages sent voluntarily to the motor nerves in the spinal cord. As the signal is received, the muscle shortens as the fibers contract, and this moves the bone.

Muscles contract and shorten by converting chemical energy from food into mechanical energy, which pulls on the bones and moves them. To do this the muscle is first stimulated by nerve impulses. Individual muscles can act only to shorten the distance between attachment points – they can pull but not push. For movement in the opposite direction to occur, another muscle must be activated.

The active body of the muscle is attached to tendons that join onto the bone. The bone is pulled across movable joints. The muscle that is predominantly responsible for a particular movement is called the prime mover. Helper muscles are called synergists. Muscles do not function alone and depend on the functioning of other parts of the body.

Tendons

Strong tendons anchor muscles to bones and also link muscles to muscles. They are made of dense, fibrous connective tissue, which is non-elastic. Some tendons are enclosed in sheaths, tube-like structures lubricated by synovial fluid.

Bursae are small, fluid-filled sacs that lie between some tendons and the bones beneath them. They are lined with synovial membrane, which secretes the synovial fluid that fills each bursa. They act as cushions against severe stress and ease the movement of the tendons.

TENDONITIS

Tendonitis and tenosynovitis are painful conditions caused by the tendon or the sheath of the tendon becoming inflamed. The problem commonly occurs in wrists, fingers, and forearms. Activities such as racket sports, or typing and word-processing, which use repetitive movements, are liable to produce this condition, popularly known as Repetitive Strain Injury (R.S.I.). Reducing the stress on muscles, tendons, and joints can help relieve and prevent these debilitating conditions.

MUSCLES

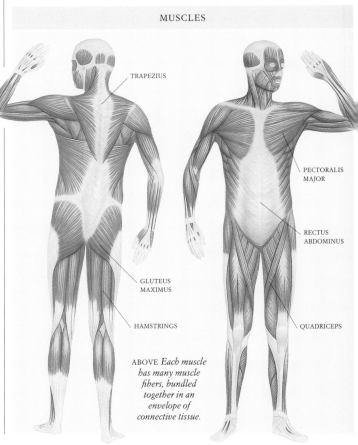

TRAPEZIUS

PECTORALIS MAJOR

RECTUS ABDOMINUS

GLUTEUS MAXIMUS

HAMSTRINGS

QUADRICEPS

ABOVE *Each muscle has many muscle fibers, bundled together in an envelope of connective tissue.*

THE BREATHING MECHANISM

The breathing mechanism consists primarily of the skeleton and muscles of the torso, which divides into the upper cavity (chest/thoracic cavity) and the lower cavity (abdomen). The chest cavity is filled almost completely by the lungs and heart, and the abdomen with the digestive tract, glands, and vital organs (viscera). Breathing is controlled by the respiratory control centers in the medulla, the hindmost segment of the brain. Under resting conditions, nervous activity in the respiratory control centers (R.C.Cs) produces a normal state and depth of breathing (12–18 respirations per minute) and in 24 hours we shift 1,850 gallons of air. The R.C.Cs are influenced by inputs from receptors located in other body areas. The cerebral cortex, the outer gray matter of the brain, can influence respiration by modifying the rate at which the nerves (neurones) "fire" in the R.C.Cs. In other words, you can change your breathing pattern during activities such as speaking, eating, and swimming, when you are able to hold your breath for short periods. This voluntary control has definite limits.

While breathing the contraction of the diaphragm makes the chest cavity longer from top to bottom. As we breathe in, the diaphragm, the large sheet of muscle shaped like a dome, which separates the thorax and the abdomen, contracts and is drawn down into the abdomen. This increases the chest cavity and the volume of the air in the lungs. Once in the lungs, air travels to the alveoli, the terminal air sacs of the lungs, where oxygen is taken up by the blood cells, and CO_2 is discharged. As we breathe out, the diaphragm is drawn upward into the chest cavity, and the volume of air in the lungs decreases. Overcontraction of the muscles of the chest restricts the movement of the ribcage.

When the muscles of the ribcage (external intercostal muscles) contract, they enlarge the chest cavity by increasing its size from front to back and from side to side, and air is drawn into the lungs. During more forceful expiration (when speaking, singing, in heavy manual work, and all sports), the internal intercostal muscles and the abdominal muscles contract and the chest cavity decreases in size from top to bottom, and air goes out of the lungs.

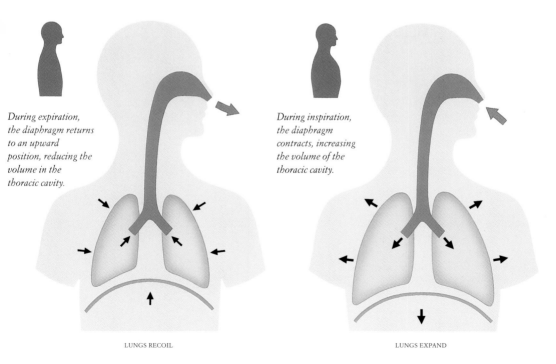

During expiration, the diaphragm returns to an upward position, reducing the volume in the thoracic cavity.

During inspiration, the diaphragm contracts, increasing the volume of the thoracic cavity.

LUNGS RECOIL

LUNGS EXPAND

Physiology: How it Works

HUMANS HAVE A *greater variety of mobility and a greater versatility of movement than animals. To move, we need energy. The Alexander Technique believes that this energy must be correctly directed. The more energy you have, the more potential damage you can do to both yourself, and other persons and things.*

GRAVITY AND WEIGHT

Although we have become accustomed to using scales to measure weight, weight is actually a variable matter of gravity working on the body. Remember the momentary feeling of weightlessness when a plane hits an air pocket? You feel as if you have left your seat. Or the feeling of your stomach staying behind you as you go up in a fast elevator? For a constant weight measurement, we need conditions that also remain constant.

The gravitational attraction of the Earth pulls every particle of the body down toward the Earth's center. At the same time, the body mass attracts every particle of the Earth, giving a resultant upward force on the earth and acting through its center. These two gravitational forces are both equal and opposite. The downward force on the body corresponds to the force responsible for the curvature of the path of unsupported objects

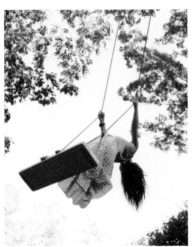

The childhood experience of playing on a swing gives a brief sense of weightlessness, demonstrating that weight is variable.

Why, man, he doth bestride the narrow world like a Colossus.

WILLIAM SHAKESPEARE:
JULIUS CAESAR

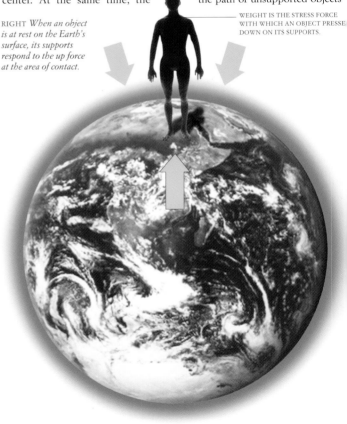

RIGHT *When an object is at rest on the Earth's surface, its supports respond to the up force at the area of contact.*

WEIGHT IS THE STRESS FORCE WITH WHICH AN OBJECT PRESSES DOWN ON ITS SUPPORTS.

and for the curvature of orbits. The upward force on the Earth corresponds to the action of the moon in raising the tide.

Professor T. D. M. Roberts is a leading authority in the neurophysiology of posture. In his book *The Neurophysiology of the Postural Mechanisms* (1967), he argues that the primary aim of the neuromuscular mechanism is to counteract the downward force of gravity. He identifies the postural reflexes as mechanisms designed to counteract the downward force of gravity with minimal effort and in such a way that we are able to realize our full physiological stature with ease and freedom: he says that the primary requirement of the neuromuscular mechanism is to make sure the head does not come into punishing collisions with its environment. The mechanism ensures that it avoids this collision by generating anticipatory preemptive actions on the basis of messages received through the kinesthetic/proprioceptive network. It preempts the danger of falling down by generating up-thrusting movements that counteract and rescue the self from the downward influence of gravity.

> Gravity allows us to stand on the ground and relate to the Earth. It is our way of knowing stability. Where do we stand, and how do we deal with space?
>
> **TESSA MARWICK,**
> **DIRECTOR OF ALEXANDER**
> **TECHNIEK CENTRUM, AMSTERDAM**

CASE STUDY

Frank Pierce Jones
Author of *Freedom to Change*

My strongest impression when A.R. Alexander first demonstrated the Technique to me was that of a mechanism working against gravity. I could not see what Alexander's brother had done, but I could perceive its effect on me. I was occupying more space; my movements were less jerky; and I had lost my customary feeling of heaviness. Whatever his procedures were, they had made a radical change in my relation to the gravitational field. The change was not an illusion, since the sensory effect lasted for the rest of the day. It was a new experience that I had neither learned nor willed. There must, I thought, be a mechanism or set of mechanisms already present – a "*physiological a priori,*" to use Magnus's term – to account for the effect.

In its relations with human beings, gravity has generally had a bad name. It is commonly thought of as a hostile force that has to be fought against and overcome. One of the most eloquent expressions of this feeling about gravity was made by the biologist D'Arcy W. Thompson. In his great book *On Growth and Form* he wrote:

Man's slow decline in stature is a sign of the unequal contest between our bodily powers and the unchanging force of gravity which draws us down when we would fain rise up. We strive against it all our days, in every movement of our limbs, in every beat of our hearts. Gravity makes a difference to a man's height, and no slight one, between the morning and the evening; it leaves its mark in sagging wrinkles, drooping mouth and hanging breasts; it is the indomitable force that defeats us in the end, which lays us on our death bed and lowers us to the grave.

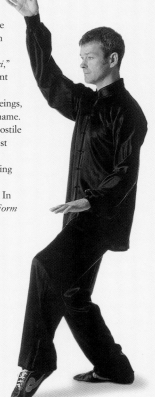

RIGHT *Practicing the Alexander Technique can create a radical re-evaluation of one's relationship to gravity, bringing about feelings of being grounded and light.*

SPIRALS

One of the basic principles upon which matter and energy are organized is spirals. Growth patterns in plants, whirlpools, whirlwinds, and the galaxies evolve and depend on spiral movements. Human anatomy reflects these universal principles. Think of throwing a ball or a discus. There is an upward thrust in the whole body that allows the arm to come around and hurl the object. This spiral spring is important in nature. Human anatomy reflects these universal principles; nothing is completely straight. All the bones, joints, and muscle structures are spirally formed. The muscular structure of the heart develops through this pattern. The foetal position of the baby, or cat curled sleeping, show spirals working. Conversely, when someone gets himself "all in a twist," you see the whole body pulling in a whirlpool of tension.

HOW DIRECTIONS AND SPIRALS RELATE

Spirals run from either side of the base of the skull. They cross the spine at the shoulder-blades and follow the ribs around to the front. Then they cross the abdomen to attach to the top of the pelvic crest.

Thinking the instruction "let your knees go forward and away" allows the two spirals connecting the legs to the torso to release. The first spiral runs from the arch of the foot, up the inner calf, through the knee to the outer thigh, around the buttocks to the sacrum and the back crest of the pelvis. The second spiral runs from the outer edge and top of

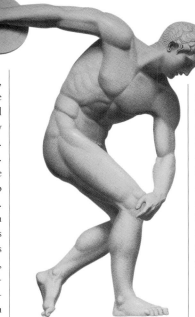

ABOVE *Thinking the instruction "let the neck be free so the head can go forward and up, and the back can lengthen and widen" allows the deep spirals that connect the head to the hips to release.*

the foot, up the outer calf, around the knee, and up the inner thigh over the front of the pelvis to attach to the front of the lumbar spine.

Thinking about the direction of widening across the upper part of the body allows the two spirals of the arm to release. The first spiral runs from the thumb and palm, up the inside of the forearm through the elbow to the back of the upper arm, then fans out from the shoulder to the head and upper back (trapezius). The second spiral runs from the little finger through the back of the hand to the back of the forearm, then through the inner upper arm to the armpit, after which it fans out and down to the lower back and sacrum.

REFLEXES

The most well-known clinical reflex is the knee-jerk. Charles Sherrington proved that in the muscles were sensitive muscle spindles, linked to the spinal cord via nerve fibers. It was the muscle spindles sending a shower of sensory impulses into the spinal cord that caused the reflex. He observed that for every action there was an equal and opposite inhibition of the action of the muscle, which would normally be its mechanical opponent. In order to allow the muscle in the front of the thigh to shorten, the muscle in the back of the thigh lengthens.

Any act... which employs a (voluntary) muscle cannot fail to enlist reflex action from it... This reflex factor is as important for the right performance of movement and posture as is the tuning of a string for the harmonious use of it in music.

Alexander said that "we do not know how we use ourselves any more than a dog or a cat knows." When it comes to physical coordination, none of us knows what we are doing. If we did, we probably wouldn't be able to do it. When Alexander said, "the right thing does itself," he was referring to a reflex process that must not be interfered with, and must not be controlled if it is going to be able to "do itself." Sherrington believed that:

This mastery of the brain over the reflex machinery does not take the form of intermeddling with reflex details; rather it dictates to a reflex mechanism "you may act" or "you may not act".

The functioning of a specific movement reflects the overall functioning of the organism. Sherrington paid tribute to Alexander's practical treatment of this issue when he said:

In urbanized and industrialized communities, bad habits in our motor acts are especially common. But verbal instruction as to how to correct wrong habits of movement and posture is very difficult. The scantiness of our sensory perception of how we do them makes it so... Mr. Alexander has done a service to the subject by insistently treating each act as involving the whole integrated individual, the whole psycho-physical man.

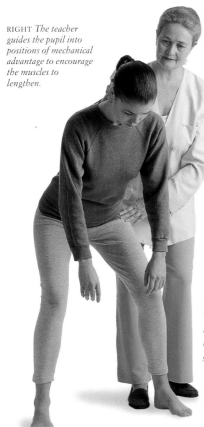

RIGHT *The teacher guides the pupil into positions of mechanical advantage to encourage the muscles to lengthen.*

MUSCLE FIBER

Muscle fibers divide into white fibers for strength, and red fibers for rhythmic movement and posture. Red fibers, though not as strong as white fibers, do not tire as quickly and are therefore ideally suited for maintaining the appropriate curve of the lower back which allows lengthening to take place.

When inadequate use is made of postural fibers, notably the deeper paraspinal muscles, then problems of posture arise. An extreme example is the experience of astronauts who, despite exercising to maintain the endurance and strength of their muscles in space, experience some atrophy that seems predominantly to affect the red fibers. Experiments with rats indicate that, following a period of time in space, their white muscle fibers were virtually unchanged, but the red fibers of their back showed both atrophy and a change in their characteristics, by which they became more like white fibers. The force of gravity is necessary to stimulate the postural fibers. Dr. David Garlick explains:

The red postural fibers, particularly of back muscles used to support the trunk, require tonic (that is, constant) nerve firing from the various sensory mechanisms stimulated by gravity (semicircular canals, stretch receptors of calf muscles, etc)... Also, stimulation to the postural fibers needs to be performed at a low level of activity, not at the higher levels of strength often used in exercises.

Five senses (hearing, sight, smell, touch, and taste) are concerned with the external environment while the sixth sense conveys signals from the muscular system. David Garlick argues that these muscle signals can be suppressed or "gated out" before reaching consciousness, and that the more we are preoccupied with the external world, the more likely we will be to shut out information from our internal world. Natural mechanisms, such as strong emotions or loud music, excite the five senses at the expense of proprioceptive information. Furthermore, our body posture and movement programs do not require continued attention, so it is common to disregard our own internal sensory feedback.

With the Alexander Technique, red muscle fibers that have changed through misuse and overuse into white fibers are gradually converted back into red fibers. This means that the appropriate balance of red and white fibers in the body is re-established through lessons in the Alexander Technique.

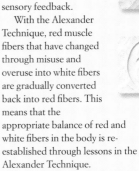

ABOVE *Sensory appreciation is the sixth sense that allows us to evaluate our limb and body position and movement.*

BREATHING

For any organism to function it needs energy. The chemical reaction that turns the food we eat into energy requires oxygen and produces carbon dioxide as a waste product. Oxygen is obtained from the air by means of the lungs. They are enclosed in the thorax, have a spongy texture, and can be expanded and compressed by movements of the thorax in such a way that air is inhaled and exhaled. As the lungs are thus ventilated, gaseous exchange of oxygen and carbon dioxide occurs between the air and the blood vessels in the lungs.

The average lung capacity of an adult is about 10 pints (5 liters), but in normal tidal breathing the exchange is only about a quarter of that. During exercise, more energy and more oxygen are required, so the capacity is increased. The thorax can never collapse completely, so there are about 3 pints (1.5 liters) of residual air that cannot be exhaled. This air exchanges carbon dioxide and oxygen by diffusion with the tidal air that comes into the lungs.

Inspiration

To inhale, the space in the thorax must be increased, causing the lungs to expand and draw in air through the nose and trachea. This is achieved by the diaphragm, the sheet of tissue separating the thorax from the abdomen. When relaxed, it is domed slightly upward. When the diaphragm is contracted, it flattens out, thereby increasing the volume of the thorax. The short intercostal muscles run from one rib to the next in a diagonal direction, away and down from the spine. When contracted they pull the ribcage upward and outward, increasing the thoracic volume.

Expiration

The lungs are essentially elastic, and once the thoracic volume is decreased, they will shrink back to their relaxed size, forcing air out again. To achieve this the diaphragm and intercostal muscles relax, allowing the diaphragm to return to its domed shape and the ribs to move downward and inward.

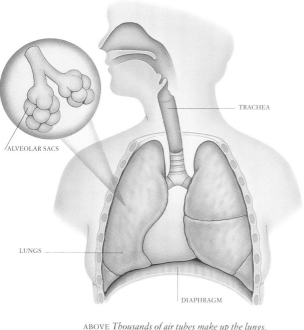

ABOVE *Thousands of air tubes make up the lungs.
The trachea branches into the bronchi, which
divide into smaller tubes called bronchioles.
These subdivide into microscopic alveolar sacs.*

ALVEOLAR SACS

TRACHEA

LUNGS

DIAPHRAGM

BELOW *Vital capacity is the largest volume
of air that can be moved in and out during
ventilation. Residual volume is the air that
remains after a forceful expiration.*

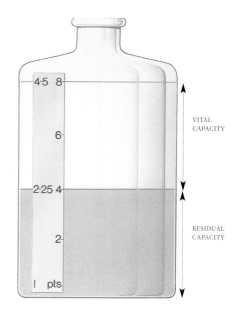

VITAL CAPACITY

RESIDUAL CAPACITY

HOW THE
VOICE WORKS

The vocal mechanism (voice) consists of three parts that need to work in coordination.

1. The Energizer

The voice needs breath to work. It is like the wind in the sails of a boat, providing the necessary energy for the boat to move forward. The efficient working of the energizer is dependent on the whole psychophysical mechanism. Posture, structure, emotion, and the situation you are in all play vital parts in how well the energizer functions.

2. The Vocalizer

Within the larynx, the vocal folds move together to make sound. This is facilitated by the muscles that attach to the laryngeal cartilage in such a way that they become more tense or relaxed. When they are tense, the voice is high-pitched; when they are relaxed, the pitch is lower.

3. The Resonators

Resonance depends on three conditions: the size of the space, or cavity; the number of openings off the cavity; and the actual structure of the walls of the cavity. The walls of a cavity correspond to the walls of a room. Sound is quite different in an empty room to one filled with furniture or people. The inside of your nose (sinus cavity), mouth, and pharynx all affect sound differently. The spaces in your face, head, throat, and upper chest are all used as resonating chambers – they are called the pharyngeal, oral, facial, and nasal cavities.

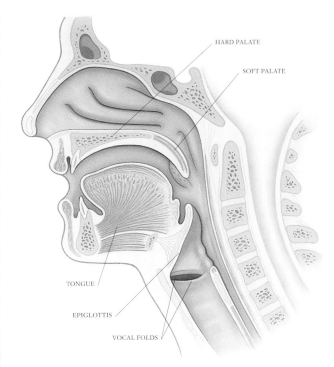

HARD PALATE

SOFT PALATE

TONGUE

EPIGLOTTIS

VOCAL FOLDS

ABOVE *The larynx (voice box) is in the pharynx (throat) and is composed of several pieces of cartilage (Adam's apple). The trachea (windpipe) extends from the larynx to the bronchi in the chest cavity.*

THE PHYSICS OF BREATHING

If gas is kept at a constant temperature, the pressure and volume are in inverse proportion or have a constant product. If air is confined at atmospheric pressure in an airtight container, there will be equal amounts of pressure acting on the outer and inner walls of the container and the differential pressure will be zero. Decreasing the volume of the container will increase the pressure inside with respect to the outside, whereas an increase in the volume of the container will decrease the pressure in the container with respect to the outside. In man, the lungs lie enclosed in the container of the airtight chest cavity (thoracic cavity) and communicate with the outside through the windpipe (trachea) and mouth (oral cavity). The structure of the chest cavity is such that its volume can be made to increase or decrease. Increase in volume of the chest cavity creates negative pressure in the lungs with respect to the outside. Consequently, air will rush into the lungs (this is called inspiration) until the inside and outside pressures are equalized. Decrease in the size (volume) of the chest cavity causes air to rush out of the lungs in the same way (this is called expiration).

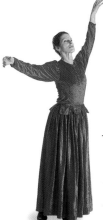

The Procedures:
Thinking in Activity

MARCUS AURELIUS SAID *that we become like our habitual thoughts. In the following procedures, we are going to look at how you can begin to change your way of doing things. Lessons in the Alexander Technique will help you to acquire the experience you need to get the most out of these procedures. This is possible because you can employ the two principles of the Alexander Technique: inhibition and direction.*

LEFT *The Alexander Technique can help us achieve grace, poise, and full creative expression of ourselves.*

Because you are unique, you will bring your own special talents and problems to every action you perform. Perhaps you will be quick to agree mentally with the principles explained in an idea, but slow to make your thoughts connect with your movements. You may be able to feel things in your body immediately, but not know how to respond to this feedback. You may be able to see the movement in your "mind's eye," but will not be able to manage the graceful rendition of your private picture. There are a few lucky people who will be able to think about, then see, hear, and feel the movement working together. This ability is commonly described as being talented, coordinated, skilled, or just plain lucky. Most of us, however, will need some help to achieve this state.

The Alexander Technique will teach you how to co-ordinate yourself more efficiently, save your energy, and boost your enthusiasm. Alexander teachers are trained to help you realize your responsibility

> The ideal condition would be,
> I admit,
> That man should be right
> by instinct;
> But since we are all too likely to
> go astray
> The reasonable thing is to learn
> from those who can teach.
>
> **SOPHOCLES: ANTIGONE**

for yourself. They guide you in the performance of everyday movements until you learn how to apply the techniques of inhibition and direction for yourself.

Trained teachers are capable of noticing when you have reverted to your old habits. Habits are hard to break, but you can, with the help of a teacher, change the way you perform everyday actions. By using your own good sense, you can begin to think about "how" you use yourself. Bringing your conscious mind to bear on any action is not going to make you lose your spontaneity. By

breaking your habitual patterns and reactions, you can make things easier for yourself.

We have therefore to see that while carrying out these procedures we do not allow improper movements, resulting from our bad habits, to occur. Sherrington states: "Breathing, standing, walking, sitting, although innate, along with our growth, are apt, as movements, to suffer from defects in our ways of doing them," Alexander originally advised practicing "before a looking glass in which to watch ourselves trying it."

We can check bad habits by observation. Alternatively, a skilled instructor maintains the head in a proper, or less twisted, position relative to the neck, while the pupil consciously inhibits the habitual movements (for example, bringing the legs toward each other while sitting down or getting up from a chair) that interfere with the proper performance of any action.

As you go through these procedures, try to be aware of your

THE MOVEMENTS

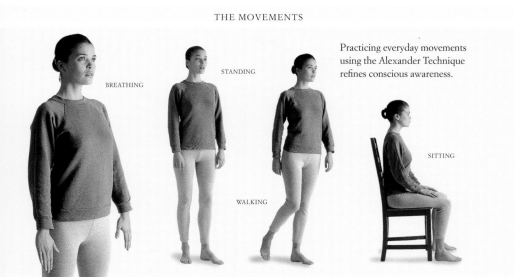

BREATHING

STANDING

Practicing everyday movements using the Alexander Technique refines conscious awareness.

SITTING

WALKING

balance and poise throughout each movement. By breaking up the procedures into steps, you will be giving yourself a chance to consider the different positions that you adopt throughout each stage of the movement. As the anthropologist, Professor Raymond Dart has said in his publication *Skill and Poise*: "The movement of an acrobat or gymnast is performed by a body that at every phase of the movement, that is the initial, intermediate and terminal positions, is in a state of mobile equipoise or balance."

> God guard me from the
> thoughts men think
> In the mind alone
> He that sings a lasting song
> Thinks in a marrow bone.
>
> **WILLIAM BUTLER YEATS:**
> **PRAYER FOR OLD AGE**

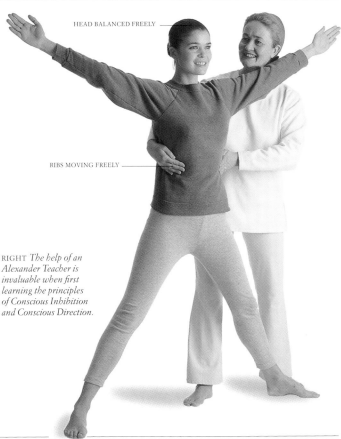

HEAD BALANCED FREELY

RIBS MOVING FREELY

RIGHT *The help of an Alexander Teacher is invaluable when first learning the principles of Conscious Inhibition and Conscious Direction.*

43

STANDING

Instead of using the legs as weight-bearing struts, think of keeping your neck free and your head going forward and up, and your back lengthening and widening. This takes the pressure off the legs so it is not necessary to brace the ankles, knees, or hips. Now let your weight go down through your heels, but don't push back on your heels. Dropping your weight releases your lower back, and your hips are free to drop back and down. Avoid squeezing your toes, bracing your knees, or stiffening your ankles. The arch of your foot should be lively. The three weight-bearing points of the foot are the heel, and the points just behind the big toe and behind the small toe forming a tripod, the arch being the top of the tripod.

You will discover how a dynamic posture emerges out of your awareness of what you do not need to do.

BELOW *The weight-bearing points of the foot include the five toe pads.*

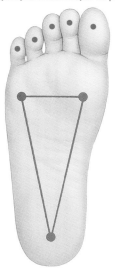

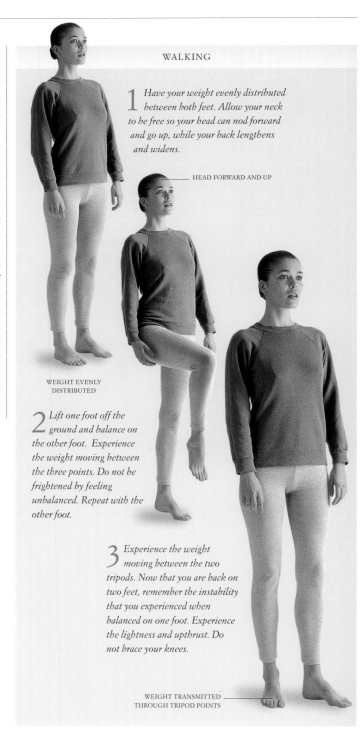

WALKING

1 *Have your weight evenly distributed between both feet. Allow your neck to be free so your head can nod forward and go up, while your back lengthens and widens.*

HEAD FORWARD AND UP

WEIGHT EVENLY DISTRIBUTED

2 *Lift one foot off the ground and balance on the other foot. Experience the weight moving between the three points. Do not be frightened by feeling unbalanced. Repeat with the other foot.*

3 *Experience the weight moving between the two tripods. Now that you are back on two feet, remember the instability that you experienced when balanced on one foot. Experience the lightness and upthrust. Do not brace your knees.*

WEIGHT TRANSMITTED THROUGH TRIPOD POINTS

WAY OF WALKING

Being able to walk in the upright position is one of the great human achievements in the long course of evolution. When walking, it is important that you maintain the poise of the body by not collapsing down into your hip joints and stiffening your legs. Walking has a natural rhythm peculiar to each of us. We often recognize someone coming toward us long before we can see their faces by their way of walking. When we are feeling well or have something to look forward to, we walk with a spring in our step, when we are ill or depressed, we become like Shakespeare's schoolboy, "creeping like snail, unwillingly to school." The fact that we can move in the upright posture requires a balancing act. Dynamic instability, fear of falling, is inherent within this relationship between gravity and uprightness. This fear can tend to make us overcompensate by using too much muscular effort.

We need to become more aware of our feet and the part they play in the way we walk. As we walk, the arches of our feet act as shock absorbers. As the weight transfers onto the foot, we make the footprint. Then the flexors of the toes contract and the back foot is actively propelled forward. We usually walk on firm, even ground, with our feet protected by shoes. Therefore there is little need for our arches to adapt to different terrain. When we begin to expose our feet to more sensations, we keep the muscles active, increasing feedback. Reflexology works on the principle that the feet represent the microcosm of the body, with all organs, glands, and other body parts laid out in a similar arrangement on the feet.

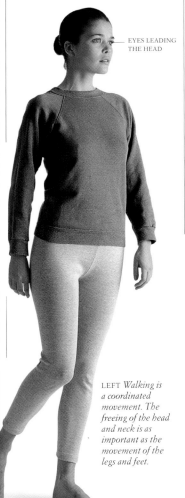

EYES LEADING THE HEAD

LEFT *Walking is a coordinated movement. The freeing of the head and neck is as important as the movement of the legs and feet.*

HEAD LEADS
BODY FOLLOWS

Your feet play a very important part in how you walk. Think of what it feels like to walk on thick carpet or soft grass, or about walking barefoot on a rough wooden floor with possible splinters. Think of walking on rough terrain, uphill, downhill, over stones. Did you tighten your toes to avoid stubbing them on the rough bits? Think about walking on the beach with burning hot sand. Did you spring onto the wet sand at the water's edge? Think of walking on icy pavements and in high-heeled shoes.

Walking only requires a small part of your available muscle power, so there is a reserve for you to use when some special action is required, such as walking upstairs, running, climbing a mountain. It is not necessary to make undue effort to walk if you are prepared to move. You need to look out and see where you want to go. The eyes lead the head and then the body moves.

WAYS TO WALK

Do
▲ Free the neck and let the head go forward and up.
▲ Free the ankle joints.
▲ Breathe out on the movement.
▲ Let the knees go forward easily.
Don't
▲ Stiffen the neck.
▲ Hold the breath.
▲ Take a big step.
▲ Let your weight sink into your hips.
▲ Let your weight roll from side to side (rolling gait).
▲ Flatten the arch of the foot.

Here comes the lady
O so light a foot
Will ne'er wear out the everlasting flint

**WILLIAM SHAKESPEARE:
ROMEO AND JULIET**

WALKING

1 *Stand equally with both feet. Breathe out and bend the knee forward. Lift up one heel, then put it back down again in the same place. Think of your spine lengthening up to your head and down to your feet. Repeat this movement with both feet in an easy rhythm on the same spot.*

2 *Let your heel come off the floor, and place your foot in front. Keep the weight still on your back foot with your front foot only slightly ahead. Be careful not to make too big a movement here.*

3 *Let your head move over your front foot and transfer your weight forward. This makes the footprint. Let the rear knee bend and the heel leave the floor. Do not move from side to side. Walk forward with an easy, flowing rhythm.*

4 *Do not stiffen your arms. Let them hang freely by your sides, swinging slightly in opposing directions to your feet. Left arm goes with the right foot, right arm goes with the left foot. The swing of your arms can make walking easier.*

WALKING UP STAIRS

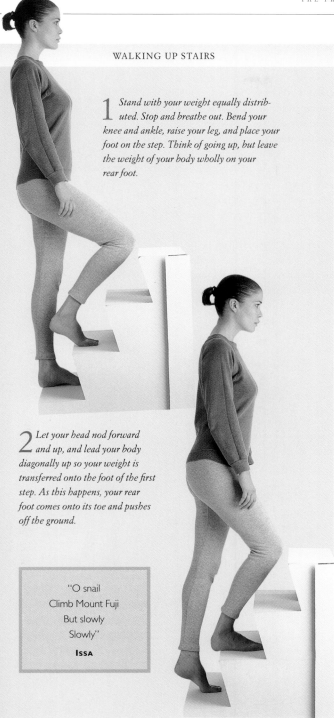

1 *Stand with your weight equally distributed. Stop and breathe out. Bend your
knee and ankle, raise your leg, and place your
foot on the step. Think of going up, but leave
the weight of your body wholly on your
rear foot.*

2 *Let your head nod forward
and up, and lead your body
diagonally up so your weight is
transferred onto the foot of the first
step. As this happens, your rear
foot comes onto its toe and pushes
off the ground.*

"O snail
Climb Mount Fuji
But slowly
Slowly"

ISSA

WALKING BACKWARD

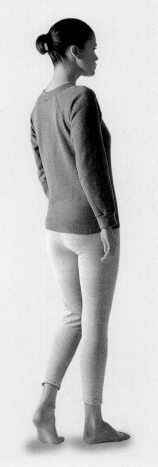

*Try a new experience of walking.
Look behind you and check that
there is room to take a few steps.
Step backward. Then place the
next foot behind you and take
another step.*

*If you are having problems with
your walking, taking a few steps
backward can break the habits that
may have been causing the problems.
Rock back before stepping forward
to remind you to stay back and not
get ahead of yourself.*

CARRYING A LOAD

Suitcases seem to get heavier and heavier as we carry them. We try to release the tension in our arms by shaking them. We try to stretch out our backs by arching backward or forward as our muscles tire. Before you lift, check you have not tightened your muscles too much.

BENDING

There are many ways of bending, and some are positively harmful. If you simply bend your knees, the large muscles of the thighs can take too much of the strain. It is important to consider whether the way

you are moving is mechanically efficient. The definition of a good machine is "one that uses minimum effort to achieve maximum efficiency." When bending, you want to reduce strain and subsequent wear and tear on the muscles, joints, and bones. If you involve your back muscles and your hip, knee, and ankle joints, you will be exercising your body and stretching all your muscles. As the muscles pull against each other, tone and suppleness are maintained. As they lengthen, the habits of contracting and shortening are reduced. Increased efficiency can lead to less discomfort and pain.

WAYS TO LIFT

Do
▲ Breathe out.
▲ Keep the thought of lengthening your muscles.
▲ Let the arms hang freely from your shoulders.
Don't
▲ Tighten your neck.
▲ Have your feet too close together.
▲ Think of going down.
▲ Set yourself into a position.
▲ Stiffen the ankles and knees.
▲ Tighten in the front muscles.

LIFTING

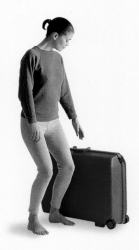 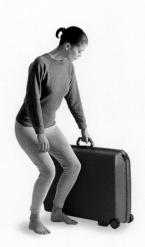 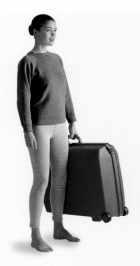

1 Free your neck and let your head go forward and up. Bend your knees and lower yourself with your arms hanging freely in front of you. Do not hold your breath.

2 Take hold of the handle of the suitcase. Do not grip it too tightly. Lift it a little way off the ground and check its weight. Put it back on the ground and breathe out. When holding the weight, allow your hips to go well back and your long back muscles to stretch.

3 Come to the standing position, bringing the suitcase with you. Be aware of maintaining your full length and try not to let your body weight be pulled over to the side of the suitcase. Begin walking in a measured rhythm.

BENDING

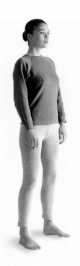

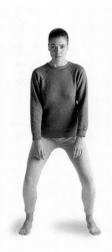

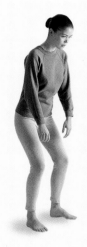

1 Stand with your feet slightly wider apart than for standing (see "Standing' page 44). Say "No" to getting ready to bend, and release your neck muscles so your head nods gently forward. Breathe out.

2 As your head nods forward, let your knees bend and your ankles bend. Your buttocks move back and down in the opposite direction by gentle lengthening and stretching of your back muscles.

3 Check your knees are pointing away from each other. When you have considered your knees going forward and away, check again that you have not stiffened your neck muscles.

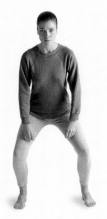

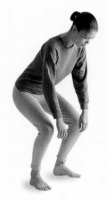

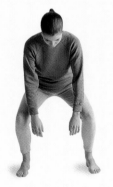

4 Allow your arms to hang freely from your shoulders so your hands are in front of your body. Do not fix into a static position, but keep the overall releasing of your muscles.

5 As your muscles lengthen and release, your ribs begin to move in and out, giving more space in the thoracic cavity and your breathing naturally deepens. Now say a whispered "Ah."

6 When you want to stand up, say "No." Free your neck and then go up until you are in the upright position. Be aware of how this way of bending has increased your muscular tone and suppleness.

SITTING

The ability to sit in the upright position is one of the most important developments in human evolution. For manual skills to develop, humans had to be in a stable position with their hands free. Most of the tool-making and tool-using activities of humans are carried out in the sitting position.

When seated, our bodies find more stability than when standing. Often we tend to sit badly, putting too much weight on our hip joints and internal organs, and creating excessive pressure on the joints and disks of our spines, and on our thighs. When we sit down to relax, it feels very comfortable at first. Taking the weight off our feet is a relief. However, as we sit, we often sag down. The longer we continue to sit in a collapsed way, the more likely we are to cause stiffness and rigidity. We have all experienced having to get up quickly to answer the door or telephone and finding that we are almost too stiff to move. We get pins and needles in our legs and feet. The reason for this is that we have moved from a collapsed, deadening posture to an active, moving one and our muscles could not respond. We can avoid this by making sitting a more conscious process and not putting so much weight down onto our joints.

Sitting in All Types of Chairs

A straight-backed chair with a flat, hard seat gives you clear feedback on your sitting position. The procedure for sitting in a soft chair is the same as for a straight-backed chair, but because the chair is soft, there

---

WAYS TO SIT

Do
- ▲ Sit on your seat/sitting bones.
- ▲ Release your ankles.
- ▲ Release your knees.
- ▲ Think of lengthening along your spine.
- ▲ Sit lightly.
- ▲ Sit with equal weight on each buttock.

Don't
- ▲ Pull your head back.
- ▲ Stiffen your neck.
- ▲ Think of going down to sit.
- ▲ Hold your breath.
- ▲ Arch your back.
- ▲ Brace your legs to get up.
- ▲ Lower yourself with your arms.
- ▲ Pull down to get up.
- ▲ Collapse in front.

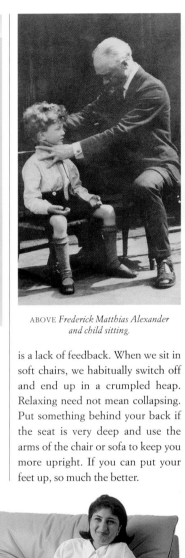

ABOVE *Frederick Matthias Alexander and child sitting.*

---

is a lack of feedback. When we sit in soft chairs, we habitually switch off and end up in a crumpled heap. Relaxing need not mean collapsing. Put something behind your back if the seat is very deep and use the arms of the chair or sofa to keep you more upright. If you can put your feet up, so much the better.

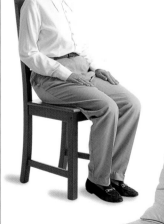

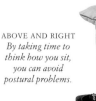

ABOVE AND RIGHT
By taking time to think how you sit, you can avoid postural problems.

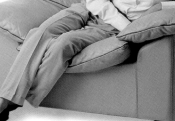

SITTING

1 Use a chair with a level seat and put your feet flat on the floor. If your chair is too low, put something on the seat. If it is too high, put something under your feet.

2 Stand in front of the chair with your feet apart and your weight evenly distributed between them. Do not stiffen your ankle joints and knees. Let your head pivot forward from the top joint and breathe out.

3 Do not think of going down into the chair, but be aware of the two-way stretch of your back muscles. Let the hinge mechanism of your hips work in order to bring your head back over the spine so that you are seated in the upright position.

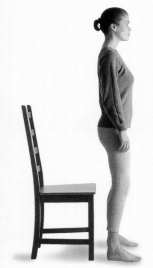
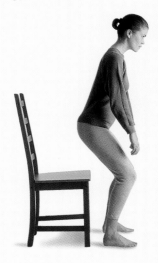
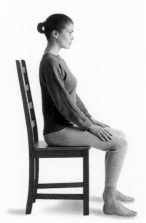

4 There are two bony projections of the pelvis called the seat bones (ischia). They are a little higher than the lower edge of your buttocks. You should be sitting on them if your pelvis is in balance.

5 Your weight should be equally divided between the front of your foot and your heel. Your feet and calves should be vertical to your knees. Do not hold yourself up rigidly as the seat of the chair is supporting your weight.

6 Make sure your feet are flat on the floor and your ankles are not stiff. Let your head lead the movement by gently nodding forward so that your body follows your head and moves up in space.

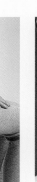
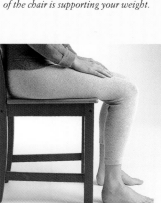
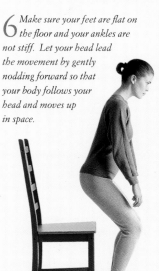

READING

The earliest books were large and heavy. People needed to use stands with sloping surfaces (lecterns) on which to rest the books. This also allowed the books to be viewed at an angle that made reading easier on the eyes. The lectern is not essential for modern books, which are not as large or heavy, but having the book at an angle to your eyes is beneficial. It allows you to see more efficiently and prevents the strain that can develop in both your neck and shoulders from looking directly downward. Resting the book on the back of a chair is a good way of improvising a lectern. When you are reading in bed, prop yourself up with pillows and bend your knees to form a natural slope on which to place your book.

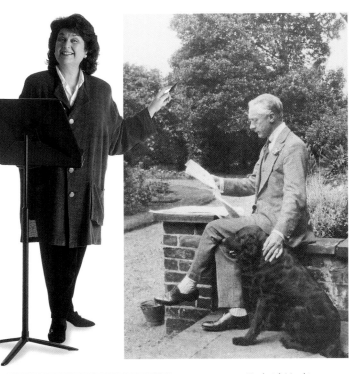

ABOVE *A lectern provides a good angle for your book.*

BELOW *Resting a book on the back of a chair is a good way of improvising a lectern.*

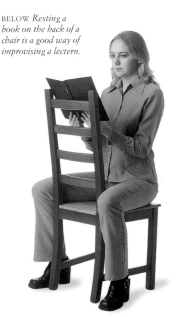

ABOVE *Frederick Matthias Alexander reading.*

BELOW *When you are sitting on a soft chair, sit well back and put pillows behind you.*

WAYS TO READ

Do
- ▲ Sit on your seat/sitting bones.
- ▲ Release your ankles.
- ▲ Release your knees.
- ▲ Think of lengthening along your spine.
- ▲ Sit lightly.
- ▲ Sit with equal weight on each buttock.

Don't
- ▲ Pull your head back.
- ▲ Stiffen your neck.
- ▲ Think of going down to sit.
- ▲ Hold your breath.
- ▲ Arch your back.
- ▲ Brace your legs to get up.
- ▲ Lower yourself with your arms.
- ▲ Pull down to get up.
- ▲ Collapse in front.

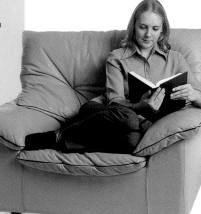

READING

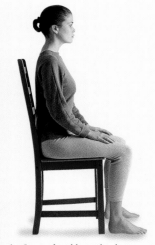

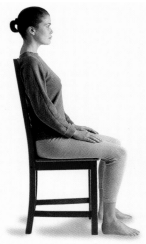

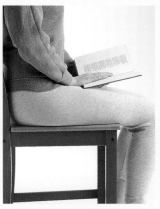

1 Sit comfortably on the chair with your feet flat on the ground. Breathe out.

2 Do not hold yourself up rigidly, but allow the back of the chair to support your back.

3 Pick up the book and rest it on your knees with your hand keeping it open and breathe out.

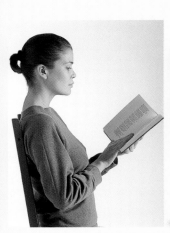

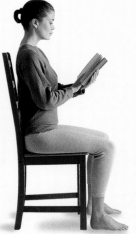

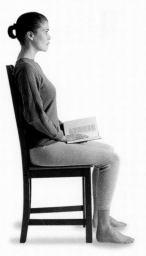

4 Lift the book by supporting the back of it with the other hand and hold it at an angle of about 45 degrees.

5 Try not to hold your breath (even when the story gets exciting).

6 Remember to put the book down on your lap and look up from the text now and then as this can stop you from overfocusing and prevent eyestrain.

HANDWRITING

Medieval manuscripts took time to write, giving pleasure both to the scribes and to those who read them. Italic writing was taught in schools, but today handwriting is not taught as carefully. Many of us type, missing out the link between forming the letters manually and the satisfaction that a well-written page gives.

Today we write with a variety of implements – pencils, fountain pens, fiber-tipped pens, and crayons. We need to consider how we use the pen in order to do it with the greatest ease. Often we create undue effort by holding the pen too tightly. It is helpful to practice picking up the pen easily and making some preliminary movements in the air before you put it to the paper to write.

A sloping surface creates a better angle for your eyes and helps to prevent you from collapsing down in front, putting undue pressure on your internal organs and breathing.

WAYS TO WRITE

Do
▲ Have a good desk height.
▲ Have a sloping surface.
▲ Take time.
▲ Get up at regular intervals.
▲ Have equipment properly set up.
▲ Keep awake.

Don't
▲ Collapse forward or hunch over.
▲ Hold your breath.
▲ Stiffen your wrists.
▲ Narrow your shoulders.
▲ Tighten your forearms.
▲ Go too fast.
▲ Grip your pen.
▲ Remain seated too long.
▲ Go into a trance.

HANDWRITING

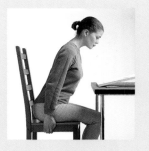

1 *Check the height of the table or desk you are going to use. You need to be able to move forward freely from the hinge joints of your hips. Point your fingers down to the ground, then take hold of the chair.*

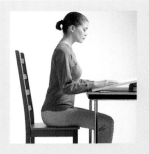

2 *Allow your head to nod forward and let your body move forward from the hinge joints of your hips. As you do this, slide your chair up closer to your desk. Breathe out and bend your arm freely at the elbow joint.*

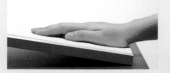

3 *Allow the muscles to flex until you can place your hand on the table. Rest for a moment, then slowly rotate your hand from the palm-down position (prone) to palm-up (supine), keeping your wrist free.*

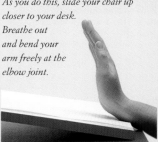

4 *Turn your hand over and flex it back from your wrist, keeping your hand straight so your fingers point directly upward.*

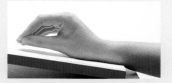

5 *Keeping them straight, flex your fingers forward from the knuckles. Rotate your thumb around so it meets the pad of your index finger. Gently bend and straighten your finger and thumb. Repeat a few times until it feels smooth and easy.*

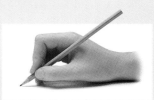

6 *Place your pen between your index finger and thumb. Hold it gently. Repeat the bending and straightening of your fingers and thumb with the pen in your hand. Put the pen to paper, take your time, and make some definite strokes.*

USING A KEYBOARD

Although we no longer need great muscular effort to push down the keys of old-fashioned typewriters, typing still causes neck aches, headaches, frozen shoulders and frustration. Much time and money is spent on designing offices that are ergonomically correct. No matter how good the design of the chair is, if the way we sit in it is poor, then the aches and pains which result from long periods of sitting will not be prevented.

As we work, we tend to lose concentration and go into a trance. Becoming aware of our breathing pattern can reduce neck strain in these situations. As the flow of air keeps the intrathoracic cavities open, more oxygen can get to our brains. This helps to keep us awake, and enables us to be more conscious of what we are doing. When we are bored, we make mistakes. Taking short breaks, even standing for a few moments, can help.

BELOW *The design and function of people using a work space is all too often ignored.*

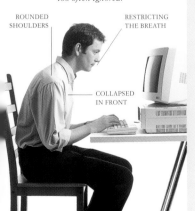

ROUNDED SHOULDERS

RESTRICTING THE BREATH

COLLAPSED IN FRONT

USING A KEYBOARD

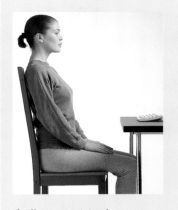
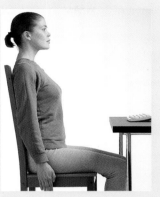

1 *Keep maintaining the two-way stretch of your back muscles. When your buttocks reach the seat, let the hinge mechanism of your hips work in order to bring your head back over the spine, so that you are seated in the upright position in the chair.*

2 *Stretch your fingers down toward the ground and breathe out*

3 *Breathe out and bend your arms freely at the elbow joints. Place your hands on the table, keeping your arms at right angles to the table. Come forward from your hips so that you are in a good position to see.*

4 *Begin as you did for writing, but this time, after flexing your hands back from your wrists, place them gently on the keyboard. When your fingers are over the keys you wish to press, say "No" to the thought of hurrying, free your neck, breathe out. Do not make undue effort and especially try not to tighten your wrists.*

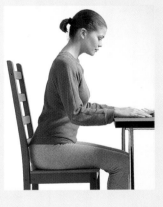

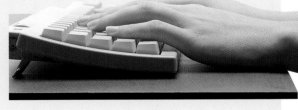

SQUATTING

Squatting is the natural way to raise and lower ourselves. Small children employ this way of getting up and down all the time, although later in life many of us lose the ability. Squatting is the simplest natural way to get close to the ground. If we did not have chairs to sit on, we would squat.

Squatting can give a good stretch to the long muscles of the back and stimulate the soft internal organs (viscera) of the body. Many may feel that it is an impossible movement, but this is only lack of use. As the general tone of your body improves, and as your ankles become freer, then squatting becomes possible.

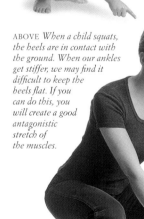

ABOVE *When a child squats, the heels are in contact with the ground. When our ankles get stiffer, we may find it difficult to keep the heels flat. If you can do this, you will create a good antagonistic stretch of the muscles.*

SQUATTING

1 *Stand with your feet slightly wider apart than for the standing procedure (see "Standing," page 44). This helps to maintain your balance when you lower yourself to the ground. Say "No" to the feeling that you will not be able to squat.*

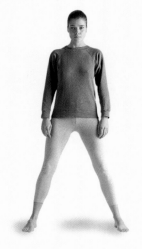

2 *Continue with these directions until you encounter any resistance in your muscles. Stop where you are and wait for a second, then see if you can continue. If you find further movement is not possible, stop where you are.*

3 *In the squatting position, allow your arms to hang freely between your knees ready for use (see "Lifting," page 57). Stay like this for as long as you feel comfortable in order to give your muscles a chance to release into the new position.*

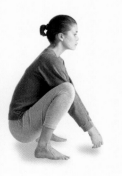

4 *When you decide to get up, think of where your head will go. It needs to move in a diagonal direction up over your feet. Do not overtighten your leg muscles.*

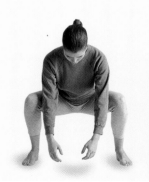

LIFTING AN OBJECT (INANIMATE)

Do you remember going to the circus and watching the clowns struggling to lift the heavy dumb-bells? Their unsuccessful attempts to move the weights were very funny. Then suddenly they were hitting each other over the head with the dumbbells, and you realized that what you had thought were huge heavy balls were actually made of foam rubber, painted to look like gray metal.

When we imagine things are going to be heavy, we will find them more difficult to lift if we get ready with too much muscular tension. Often we expect things to be heavy so we get ready by taking a deep breath and then holding it. This tension in the body will not help.

When you grasp an object, the shape of your hand needs to change. The position that the hand naturally assumes is called the "position of function" of the hand. When the muscles and joints of the hand are in a state of equilibrium, promoting muscular efficiency, then we can grasp an object with minimal effort. Two things can help you prepare for lifting. Remember inhibition, and say "No" and remember to give your directions. Try not to expect the task to be difficult or impossible, then the lifting procedure can become a little easier if you move freely. Your body weight can become an effective counterbalance – overstiffening our muscles and holding our breath can cause defeat before we have begun.

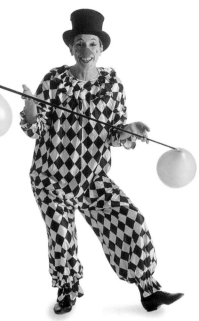

ABOVE *Don't make undue effort… it is not as heavy as you think.*

LIFTING AN INANIMATE OBJECT

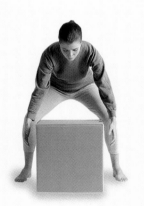

1 *Before you lift, pause for a moment and ask yourself whether you are generating unnecessary effort in preparing to lift.*

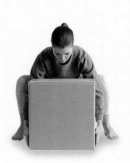

2 *Being careful not to grip too tightly, take hold of the object. When you grasp an object, the handle follows the life line of the hand. Bend your knees and lower yourself and take hold of the object. Lift it a little way off the ground and check the weight of it.*

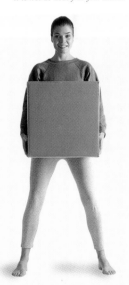

3 *You may find that the move was easier than you had expected. By not stiffening your arms, you have not interfered with your breathing.*

LIFTING AN OBJECT (ANIMATE)

When we have to lift a baby or a child, so often we hold our breath. Because we are frightened we might lose our grip, we tend to hold on too tightly. Our hands must change shape, but not to the extent that they become claws and by their excessive tension frighten the baby. We need to balance the weight of our body against the moving weight of the living object we are trying to lift. Because we feel we need to hold the baby close to us, we often create too much tension in our arms and shoulders. We can hold someone freely yet securely without tightening. Support and a feeling of security are given to the child through the feelings in our body.

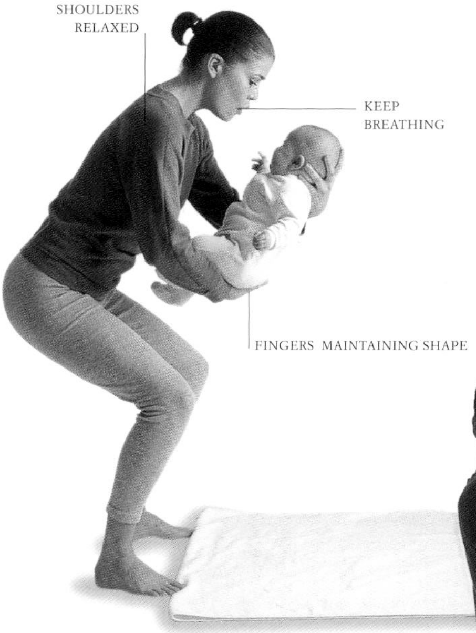

SHOULDERS RELAXED

KEEP BREATHING

FINGERS MAINTAINING SHAPE

LEFT *In order to lift a child safely, it is important to remain relaxed; otherwise, the tension in our bodies will be communicated to the child.*

LIFTING AN ANIMATE OBJECT

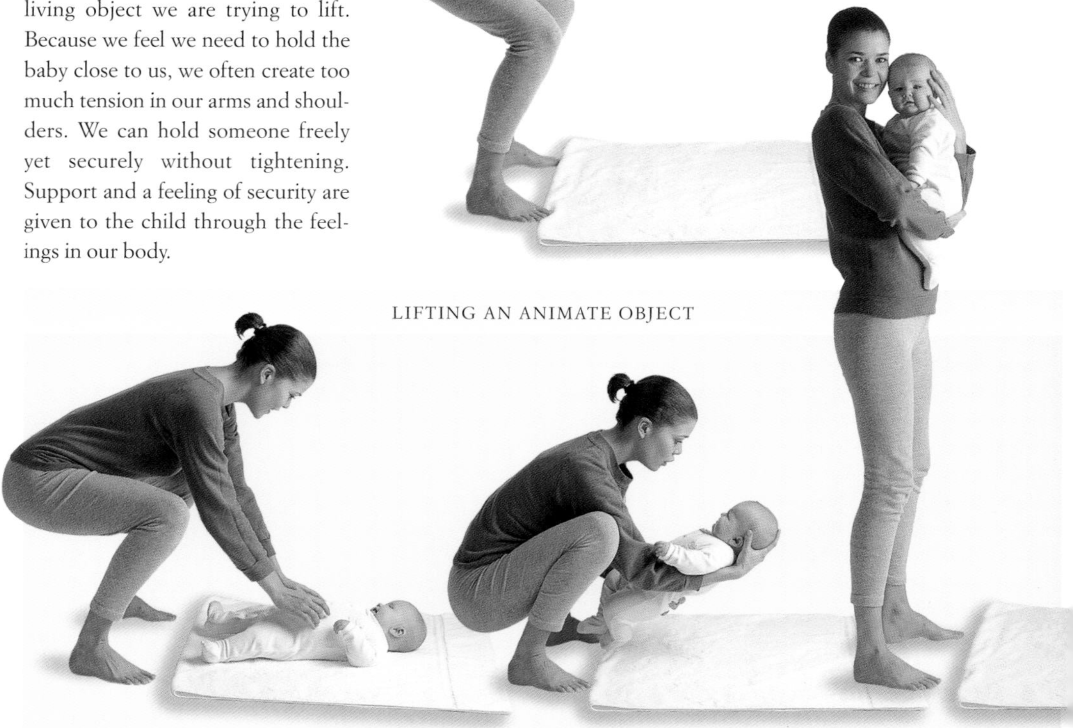

1 *Before you lift, pause for a moment and ask yourself whether you are generating unnecessary effort in preparing to do so. Pay attention to your neck and let your head go forward and up.*

2 *Being careful not to grip too tightly, take hold of the object. Lift it a little way off the ground and register the weight of it. When holding the weight close to your body, allow your hips to go well back and your long back muscles to stretch.*

3 *You may find that the move was much easier than you had expected. By not stiffening your arms, you have not interfered with your breathing or pulled down in front causing pressure on your internal organs.*

REACHING UP WITH THE ARMS

We need to be able to reach up with our arms without incurring pain or even injury. We can strain our shoulders, and stiffness can result if we use our arms wrongly. If this misuse is persistent, "frozen shoulder" can be the result.

The flexible design of the shoulder leads to common problems in the joints and muscles. The medial end of the clavicle, or collar-bone, is the firm cartilaginous attachment fastening the shoulder girdle to the

trunk. The clavicle runs the width of the shoulders and of the upper body, and is at the center of movement of the arms. The muscles provide support for the arms and allow for the movement of the hand. When operating to raise the arm, these muscles can easily overtighten, and inflammation or tendonitis can result. This painful condition can make raising the arms even a small degree almost impossible (see page 34).

WAYS TO REACH

Do
▲ Free the neck.
▲ Breathe out.
▲ Drop the shoulders.
▲ Lengthen the fingers.

Don't
▲ Lift the shoulders.
▲ Hold the breath.
▲ Brace the knees.
▲ Overextend the elbow joint.
▲ Drop the head back.

RIGHT *Like a child, prepare to reach for something by using your eyes, without pulling your head back.*

REACHING UP

1 *Rotate your arms so your palms are facing forward. This anatomical position helps your shoulder girdle to release.*

2 *Turn your hand around so your palm is facing backward. Your shoulder girdle should move freely with your arm as an extension of your head, neck, and back.*

3 *Look up and begin to lift the arm by allowing your pointing finger to lead the movement. Try not to sway.*

4 *Raise the other arm so both arms are reaching up. Be careful not to lift your shoulders, and do not brace your knees, arch your back, or hold your breath.*

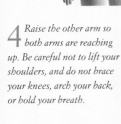

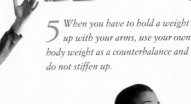

5 *When you have to hold a weight up with your arms, use your own body weight as a counterbalance and do not stiffen up.*

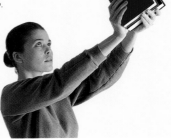

LYING DOWN
(SEMI-SUPINE)

Lying down is one of the quickest and simplest ways of allowing our bodies to come back into shape. This procedure has beneficial effects. It allows the spine to de-rotate and lengthen, and brings the head into a more forward position relative to the neck. In the supine position with knees bent, the pelvis can tilt backward and the lumbar curve flattens out. The spinal and abdominal muscles can release undue tensions, allowing gravity to have a beneficial effect on the diaphragm (see Breathing, page 40) and the ribcage to work more effi-ciently. A deeper breathing pattern happens, and the whole system calms down.

Without the fear of falling, the inherent elasticity of the body has a chance to reassert itself. If you lie down for ten to fifteen minutes each day, you will find that it makes an appreciable difference.

LYING DOWN

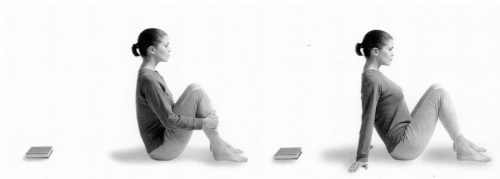

1 Put a book or some other support under your head. This needs to be at least 2in/5cm high on the floor. Sit on the floor in front of the book or other support and breathe out.

2 Allow your spine to roll down onto the floor until the back of your head is on the book. Be careful that your neck is free and your head is not jammed against the book. Too few books will reduce the natural curve of the neck, and too many could push your chin onto your chest and restrict breathing.

3 Bend your knees and bring your feet near to your buttocks. You need to have your knees bent but not strained, so your lower back is not arched but is in contact with the floor. Place your hands on your lower ribs, just above your waist.

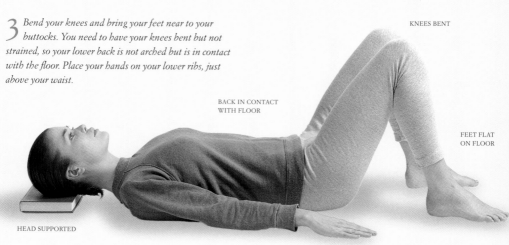

KNEES BENT

BACK IN CONTACT
WITH FLOOR

FEET FLAT
ON FLOOR

HEAD SUPPORTED

BENEFITS OF LYING DOWN

▲ Releases muscles and joints.
▲ Takes pressure off spine.
▲ Releases diaphragm giving more rib movement.
▲ Allows for more regular breathing.
▲ Gives digestive release.

▲ Frees neck muscles.
▲ Takes pressure off eyes.
▲ Jaw releases.
▲ Unclenches the hands.
▲ Gives time to think and become more conscious.

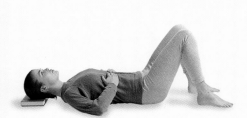

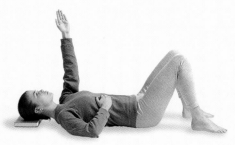

4 As you lie in this semi-supine position, allow your whole back to be in contact with the floor. Be aware of the nine, weight-bearing parts of the back – the head, the shoulders, the elbows, the hips (pelvic crests), and the feet. If you stop tightening your muscles unnecessarily, the ribs move more freely to allow the air to come in and out.

5 After about ten minutes, you will often find that your breathing has changed. When you begin to think about getting up, remember to take your time. Slowly raise one arm above your body so your fingers are pointing directly upward and then look to one side.

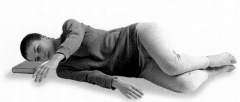

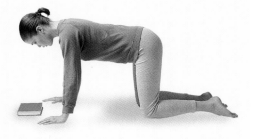

6 Let your arm lead your body so that you roll over onto your side. Stop and breathe out and check that you have not stiffened your neck or begun to overcontract your stomach muscles.

7 Move onto your hands. Rock forward and backward, allowing your head to lead your body forward. Say "No" to the idea of standing up. Bring one foot forward and put it in front of you. Allow your head to nod forward and your weight to move forward from the hips until you begin to move diagonally upward until you are standing.

CRAWLING

Crawling is one of the important stages in human development. Returning to being on all fours allows the head to move in the same direction as the spine, as is the case with animals. When an animal wants to move forward, the head leads and the body follows. If the back sags down, you will not be able to move forward easily. In order for the movement to happen, you have to allow your back to rise up. Some babies, who move from creeping to bottom bouncing, omitting the crawling stage, can have problems with growth and development later on (see pages 74–77).

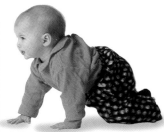

ABOVE *Crawling is one of the important stages in our development.*

CRAWLING

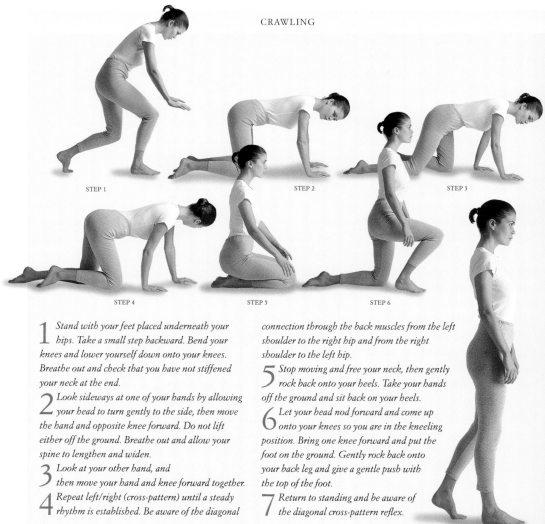

STEP 1

STEP 2

STEP 3

STEP 4

STEP 5

STEP 6

1 *Stand with your feet placed underneath your hips. Take a small step backward. Bend your knees and lower yourself down onto your knees. Breathe out and check that you have not stiffened your neck at the end.*

2 *Look sideways at one of your hands by allowing your head to turn gently to the side, then move the hand and opposite knee forward. Do not lift either off the ground. Breathe out and allow your spine to lengthen and widen.*

3 *Look at your other hand, and then move your hand and knee forward together.*

4 *Repeat left/right (cross-pattern) until a steady rhythm is established. Be aware of the diagonal connection through the back muscles from the left shoulder to the right hip and from the right shoulder to the left hip.*

5 *Stop moving and free your neck, then gently rock back onto your heels. Take your hands off the ground and sit back on your heels.*

6 *Let your head nod forward and come up onto your knees so you are in the kneeling position. Bring one knee forward and put the foot on the ground. Gently rock back onto your back leg and give a gentle push with the top of the foot.*

7 *Return to standing and be aware of the diagonal cross-pattern reflex.*

STEP 7

WEIGHT-BEARING POINTS

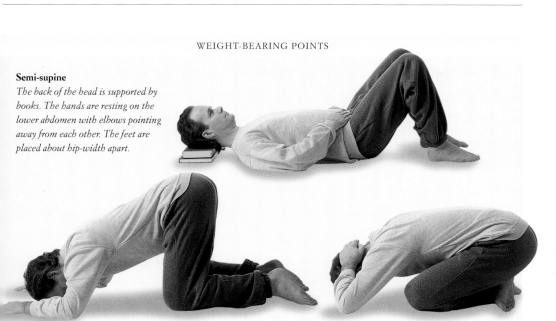

Semi-supine
The back of the head is supported by books. The hands are resting on the lower abdomen with elbows pointing away from each other. The feet are placed about hip-width apart.

Pentidpedal
The forehead, elbows, and knees are on the floor. The center of the forehead is in contact with the ground.

Crouch
The hairline of the head contacts the ground. The fingers wrap around the base of the neck.

All-fours
The weight of the body is supported by the hands underneath the shoulders and the knees underneath the hips.

WAYS TO CRAWL

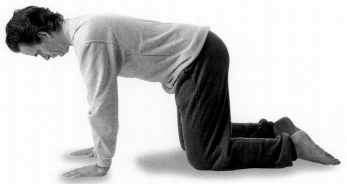

Do
▲ Keep your eyes looking downward.
▲ Remember to rotate your head sideways before moving.
▲ Let your feet trail behind you.

Don't
▲ Arch the back.
▲ Let the back sag down.

MAKING SOUNDS

The Alexander Technique grew out of the problem that Frederick Matthias Alexander had when he tried to make sounds. As a result of formulating his Technique, he found a new way to use his voice. One of the procedures that enabled him to do this was the Whispered "Ah." All voice teachers and singing teachers, including Alexander, have always valued the sound "Ah" as a measure of the effectiveness of the voice. The old singing masters understood that the ability to vocalize "Ah" was an important aspect of correctly vocalizing the other vowels. In order to produce a vowel you need a constant, unbroken stream of air. Consonants, on the other hand, interrupt this stream of air and momentarily stop the sound by using the lips, tongue, and teeth to block the air. If you can speak or sing a good, open "Ah," then the other vowels can become more open and free.

> There is a kind of voice that accords with the ear not so much by its volume but by its quality.
>
> **QUINTILIAN VI (III)**

Whispering occurs when the vocal folds do not close along their entire length. Normally, we use our voices for speaking and are much less familiar with the whispered tone. Problems can be covered up by the spoken tone, and underlying problems in vocal functioning can be revealed when "Ah" is said in a whisper. Choosing to whisper the vowel "Ah" gives you the chance to break your usual habits of vocalizing. Combining "Ah" with whispering was an inspired procedure developed by Alexander. This procedure, which allows you control of the outbreath by whispering "Ah," is one that will repay daily practice. It can increase your length of breath and strengthen your voice. This exercise can also calm you down.

As part of this procedure, think of something funny that makes you want to smile or laugh. This has the physiological effect of lifting the soft palate, livening the facial muscles, and giving a message to the diaphragm to release. As tension in the jaw and face release, saliva is secreted. This helps to prevent your mouth from drying out.

Putting the tongue against the back of your lower teeth helps you stop retracting the back of the tongue and constricting the throat, and creates an antagonistic pull in that strong muscle. The tongue is the only muscle in the whole body connected directly to a bone (hyoid bone) and exhibits a persistent tendency to overtighten and retract, not only restricting the air flow, but creating a strained vocal tone.

BELOW *The voice wheel is a way of visualizing the smooth flow of air necessary to good vocal tone.*

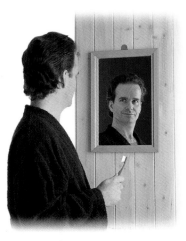

ABOVE *Take time each day to practice the whispered "Ah" in front of a mirror.*

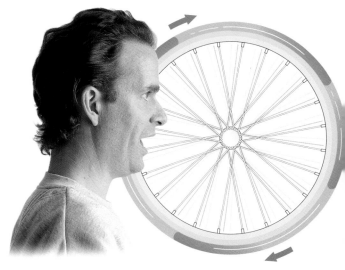

THE WHISPERED "AH"

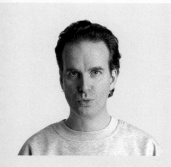

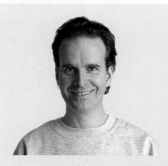

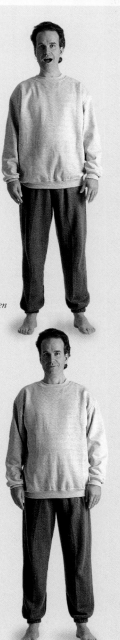

1 *Blow the air out through your mouth. Do not stiffen your neck or tighten and pull down as you exhale. Allow the air to return through your nose. Repeat.*

2 *Think of something funny that makes you want to smile or laugh. This is a very important part of this procedure and needs to be practiced. It is a simple instruction, but sometimes people do not have the ability.*

3 *Give your directions to free your neck and let the head go forward and up. The movement of the ribcage should be sufficient to generate widening in the whole torso. Do not tighten the abdominal muscles or pull down in the upper chest.*

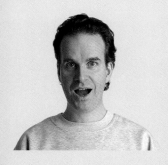

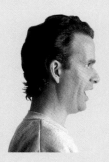

4 *Put the tip of your tongue against the back of your lower teeth. This is a preventive measure to help you stop retracting the back of the tongue and constricting the throat.*

5 *Open your mouth by allowing the jaw to drop forward and down. Do not let the weight of your head drop back and down. Say "Ah" in a whisper.*

6 *When you have come to the end of your breath, close your mouth and allow the air to come back in through your nose. As soon as the air has returned, repeat the procedure.*

THE STAR – EXPANSION THROUGH EXPIRATION

The voice cannot function to optimum capacity when the body is contracted. Taking and maintaining your full height allows the voice to work fully, preventing a strangled sound.

The star procedure encourages you to fill your total space and experience your full vocal tone.

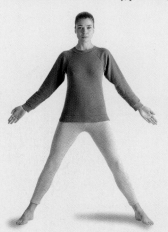

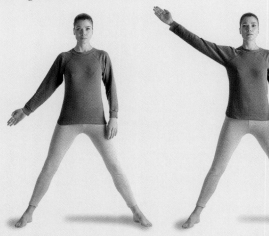

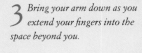

1 *Stand with your feet hip-width apart and allow your head to nod forward and up. Rotate your arms so your hands face forward.*

2 *Think of your fingers drawing your right arm up until it is at a 45° angle. Let your shoulder release down. Think of your weight going down through your left leg.*

3 *Bring your arm down as you extend your fingers into the space beyond you.*

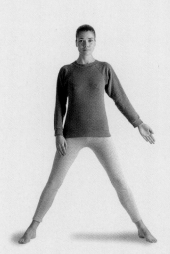

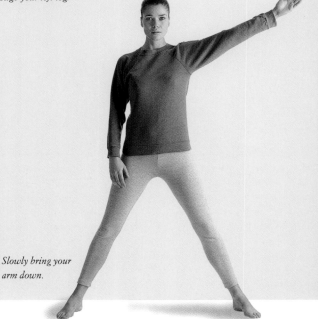

4 *Repeat Step 2, using the left arm and right leg.*

5 *Slowly bring your arm down.*

NATURAL SUPPORT

The star procedure helps you to experience how important it is to release and lengthen through the body in order to engage the supporting musculature. If too much effort is required of the abdominal muscles, the voice is blocked; if too little effort is made, there will not be enough energy to motivate the voice. Lengthening and widening helps the postural muscles to create a two-way stretch in the body, which helps the abdomen to contract appropriately.

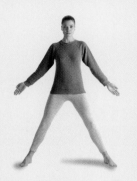 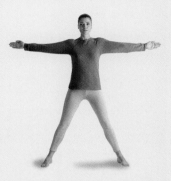 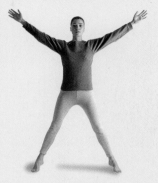

1 As you direct the weight of the body down through your feet, direct the fingers of your hands toward the ground. Rotate your arms so your hands face forward.

2 As you direct your fingers into the space beyond your reach, raise your arms to the horizontal. Release your shoulders as you reach with your fingers into the space beyond you.

3 Breathe out on the blowing sound. Close your mouth and let the air return through your nose. Repeat three times. Bring your arms down.

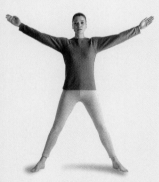 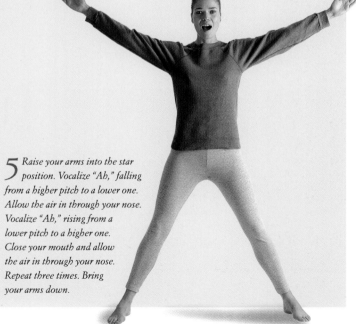

4 Raise your arms. Say "Ah" in a whisper. Repeat three times. Bring your arms down. Hum "mmm," falling from a higher pitch to a lower one. Allow the air in through your nose. Now hum "mmm" again, this time raising from a lower pitch to a higher one. Allow the air in through your nose. Repeat three times. Bring your arms down.

5 Raise your arms into the star position. Vocalize "Ah," falling from a higher pitch to a lower one. Allow the air in through your nose. Vocalize "Ah," rising from a lower pitch to a higher one. Close your mouth and allow the air in through your nose. Repeat three times. Bring your arms down.

The Procedures of Professor Dart

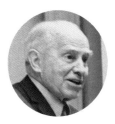

PROFESSOR RAYMOND DART

Both frederick alexander and Professor Dart came from pioneering stock in Australia. They had natural curiosity and persistence, a talent for asking unusual questions and endeavoring to answer them, and a personal need (Dart had a disabled son) which meant they had to find some practical way to help themselves. They both decided on the path of re-education: rather than learning something new, they were rediscovering something forgotten.

When he was living and working in South Africa, Dart, along with his two children, had lessons in the Alexander Technique. His son suffered spasms, and Dart dearly wished for his coordination and quality of life to improve. As an anthropologist, Dart already had extensive knowledge of man's progression to upright posture. He later wrote, "Perhaps the richest comedy presented by the evolutionary process is that creatures in nature designed to have perfect posture and vision should today represent a picture of bespectacled decrepitude."

By starting on the floor, he began to explore movement with no fear of falling. He made notes daily as he localized creaks, aches and other sensations, and became more aware of the weight-bearing body parts.

He warned that some people who try out this procedure may see the movements as "ludicrous, because they are infantile."

Lying on your back, side, or front gives enormous sensory input through the skin, stimulating your sensory "map" of yourselves. Touching surfaces can become pleasurable, as this "wakes up" the sensory nervous system.

THE MOVEMENTS

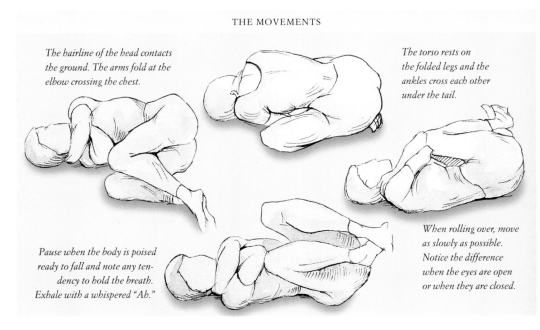

The hairline of the head contacts the ground. The arms fold at the elbow crossing the chest.

The torso rests on the folded legs and the ankles cross each other under the tail.

Pause when the body is poised ready to fall and note any tendency to hold the breath. Exhale with a whispered "Ah."

When rolling over, move as slowly as possible. Notice the difference when the eyes are open or when they are closed.

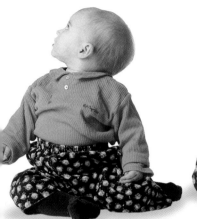

Twisting action can only occur by differentiated action between flexor and extensor action in several body segments.

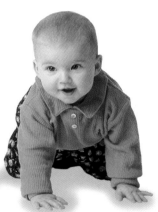

The first two vertebrae (atlas and axis) are built to allow both nodding movements of the skull on the atlas...

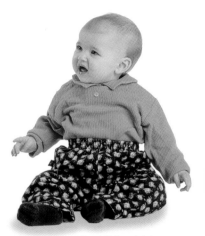

...and rotational (left and right swinging movements) of the skull and atlas upon the axis.

USE BOTH SIDES –
JEAN CLARK

While experimenting with these movements, Dart heard as muscles let go of the joints. Dart describes this as the:

> *...capacity of the synovial fluid to form gas bubbles, and the subsequent physical modifications in the quality and surface tension of the synovial fluid, enables joints, which for years have moved little if at all, to assume gradually, or even rapidly, the mobility they were fashioned to experience.*

When crawling, by exploring moving one limb at a time, first one side, then the other in a slow progression, we notice that when we want to move faster, our opposite limbs move in a cross-pattern fashion. Dart observed: "I continually discover my own faulty techniques to lie in passing too rapidly over basic essentials and rushing ahead to performance of stardom."

From crawling we can explore the transition backward and upward, one leg extended out to the side, so we can arrive at a sitting position, balancing on our seat bones. As babies this is our first experience of being upright unaided. We can explore both variations to left and right with the opposite legs extended and flexed, one rotation seeming easier for us than the other. This is because we have a dominant side related to our preferred hand and, if overindulged, over the years we begin to develop twists. We have two interwoven spiral sheets of trunk musculature directly attached to the skull: when both spirals are working in a balanced way, there is general lengthening and widening; when not, there will be scoliosis. Dart always advocated using both sides of the body and both sides of the brain, so as not to become too habituated to using only our preferred and therefore biased side.

When in a semi-supine position, we can explore movements of arms and hands by resting the backs of the arms and hands on the floor, and stroking the backs of the hands on the floor, moving from the wrist and then extending this flippering action to a movement of the whole limb from the shoulder, or the lower arm from the elbow. We can then roll onto our side, looking for a spot to place our farther hand, and then bring ourselves up and over onto our hands and knees again. From this quadruped position, we can explore being on five, weight-bearing points in a form of Muslim prayer (see page 63). With this extra head contact, we can release any unnecessary tightening in our armpits and thus open up our shoulders: "Relaxation of the unwanted muscles is the key to skilled performance."

Education

"TO COME INTO possession of intelligence is the sole human title to freedom. The spontaneity of childhood is a delightful and precious thing, but in its original naïve form it is bound to disappear. Emotions become sophisticated unless they become enlightened, and the manifestation of sophisticated emotion is in no sense genuine self-expression. True spontaneity is henceforth not a birthright, but the last term, the consummated conquest of an art – the art of conscious control, to the mastery of which Mr. Alexander's book so convincingly invites us."

John Dewey, Introduction to Man's Supreme Inheritance

The Alexander Technique grew out of the experience of one man's search to help himself. It is a means of re-educating ourselves so we can learn more easily, and retain and use what we learn. Education is a continuing process of asking questions.

"How do we work?"

"Could I be more productive?"

"Am I doing things that are limiting myself and others?"

These are the ways in which we can begin to explore our potential. The life journey that begins in the womb, through birth, babyhood, childhood, work, family life, and old age can be helped by the Alexander Technique.

The essential starting point for education is giving a child conscious control and, with it, poise. Without that poise, which is a result aimed at by neither the old nor the new methods of education, he will always be cramped and distorted by his environment. For although you may choose the environment of a nursery or a school, there are few indeed who are free to choose their desired environment in the world at large. But give the child poise and the reasoned control of his physical being, and you will fit him for any and every mode of life; he will have wonderful powers of adapting himself to the circumstances and environment in which he finds himself.

> Knowledge is experience; everything else is simply information.
>
> **ALBERT EINSTEIN**

> Everything that makes our language unique [and us human] flowed from the simple capacity to impose a delay between a signal, a message, or an event that we experience and our reaction or response to it.
>
> **JACOB BRONOWSKI**

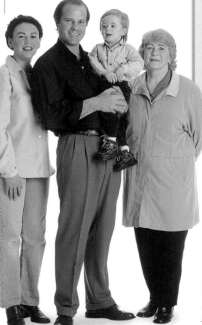

LEFT *The Alexander Technique can help everyone through their life's journey – from infants to elderly people.*

PREGNANCY AND BIRTH

ILANA MACHOVER

Pregnancy brings with it far-reaching changes in the woman's body and psyche, which affect body use and are in turn affected by it. Backache, tension, and varicose veins are common complaints. The sooner a pregnant woman begins her lessons in Alexander Technique, the better she will be able to cope with the changes of pregnancy and alleviate the complaints. The Technique can also make a crucial contribution to achieving natural childbirth.

Childbirth is a very finely tuned involuntary process. It is regulated by signals exchanged between the mother's brain and the rest of her body. The contractions of the uterus are controlled by the secretion of the appropriate hormones during each of the three phases of labor: dilation of the cervix, birth, and afterbirth of the placenta. But this process can easily be disrupted (or halted all together) by inappropriate psychological, physical, and chemical inputs. Dramatic change in the laboring woman's environment, pressure of other people around her, or continuous monitoring can all cause anxiety – and anxiety releases wrong hormones.

Any end-gaining behavior in this process is self-defeating, since the mother cannot control directly her autonomous nervous system and her hormonal balance. During the first stage of labor the dilation of the cervix happens by itself, and the woman only needs to allow the process to proceed. With each contraction, by moving in a relaxed way and agreeing to accept the pain, she can help herself to cope.

During labor it is very difficult for the unprepared woman to accept that the pain of the contractions is "normal." For the majority of women, this is the most severe pain they have ever experienced. Our society does not teach us to tolerate pain, and we are used to taking pain-killing drugs. However, these derail the natural birth process by masking the body's signals and blocking their pathways; this often makes further intervention necessary, leading to forceps or caesarean deliveries. To accept labor pain as normal, we have to understand its role: labor pain is not pathological, but functional.

CRAWLING IMPROVES COORDINATION

Crawling as taught in an Alexander Technique lesson is very beneficial during pregnancy and is a good preparation for childbirth. It helps to calm you down and control minor aches and pains. A few minutes every day will make you feel great:

1. Start by kneeling on all fours.
2. Take one small step forward on diagonally opposite limbs, say right hand and left knee, then left hand and right knee.

3. With the head leading, crawl, and let your body's weight shift to the limbs that were in front, and are now stationary.
4. Crawl slowly and rhythmically.
5. After crawling, stay for a while on all fours and gently rock the body to and fro.

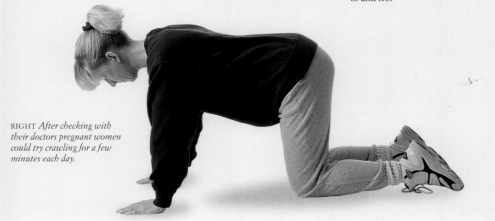

RIGHT *After checking with their doctors pregnant women could try crawling for a few minutes each day.*

Conscious Control of Pain

In this the Alexander Technique can be of enormous help. Through inhibition and direction (see page 10) we can stop our habitual reaction to pain. Instead of flexing, tensing, and pulling our heads back and down (followed by other symptoms of panic attack), we can consciously and voluntarily undo the involuntary muscle tension. We can learn to exercise conscious control over our posture and movement, giving us an indirect conscious way of affecting the hormonal balance.

This is far from easy, since the startle reflex is so often activated. We acquire the habit of going into this startle mode whenever we are stimulated to movement.

> This triumph is not to be won in sleep, in trance, in submission, in paralysis, or in anesthesia, but in a clear, open-eyed reasoning, deliberate consciousness, and apprehension of the wonderful potentialities possessed by mankind, the transcendent inheritance of a conscious mind.
>
> **F.M. ALEXANDER: MAN'S SUPREME INHERITANCE**

Consequently there is a lot of unnecessary muscle tension in most of us most of the time, especially during movement. It takes time to re-educate the body and replace habit-

ual patterns of tension with those of release. But having learned to move in her daily life without interfering with the primary control, a woman in labor can apply this skill during contractions. There is no need to be athletic or to perform complicated positions or exercises, which may only enhance patterns of tension and misuse, and encourage an attitude of end-gaining (see page 24).

Undoing the habits of a lifetime takes careful preparation. When pregnant women have lessons in the Alexander Technique, they are preparing for "Eutokia," which in classical Greek means "a happy, relaxed childbirth." It is now widely accepted that a woman should move freely and stay upright during her labor. The dynamic posture of bending (see page 49) is one of the best stances during pregnancy and is particularly advantageous during labor. In this position, as the mother leans forward, her abdominal wall becomes a kind of hammock for the baby, while the tilt of her pelvis makes more space for the baby's head to enter the pelvic brim; thus the baby is encouraged to move into the optimal position for birth. At the same time, the force of gravity – the weight of the baby – aids contractions and makes them stronger and more efficient. To soothe the pain, it is important to be able to move freely, so during labor this posture ought to be used in a dynamic way: the woman can maintain her primary control while shifting her weight from one leg to the other, either on her own or supported by her partner.

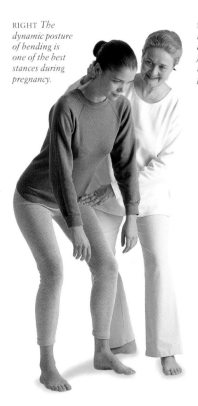

RIGHT *The dynamic posture of bending is one of the best stances during pregnancy.*

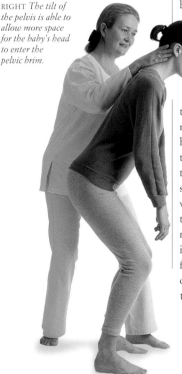

RIGHT *The tilt of the pelvis is able to allow more space for the baby's head to enter the pelvic brim.*

The Pear Movement

Ilana Machover, who runs classes in Eutokia, says: "Since many women find it helpful to go on all fours during labor, I looked for a way of making this stance more dynamic and integrating it with the principles of the Alexander Technique."

Salivation

Salivation is one of the means that can be used to achieve a relaxed state of mind and body. The body of woman in labor gets a signal that a contraction is about to begin. At this moment she should first think of a smile and allow her mouth to become wet. Thinking of something funny may help to produce a smile, releasing the tension in the jaws and face. This loosens the pressure on the salivary glands and causes them to secrete.

This is a preventive measure, which will stop the mouth from becoming too dry. Dryness of the mouth is a symptom of a panic attack. If this should occur, the practice of the whispered "Ah" is very useful.

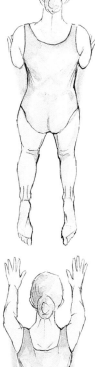

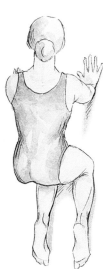

1 *The woman is on all fours and with her head leading, her body describes the shape of a pear parallel to the floor. This shape echoes the outline of the uterus.*

2 *The pear movement is useful in encouraging her to free her joints and prevent tension from accumulating, especially in the shoulders, arms, and lower back.*

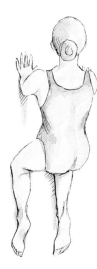

3 *With her neck free and her head leading the movement, her back lengthens and widens, so it does not sag and create tension in the lumbar area.*

GROWTH AND DEVELOPMENT OF THE CHILD

"Prevention Is Better than Cure." We should try to give children a supportive atmosphere, free from stress, in which they have time to learn about inhibition and direction, and to practice these procedures. As babies they had "I want" as a basis for behavior. As they grew up, this was replaced by what their parents, teachers, or peer pressure wanted – how they should behave and what they should do led to a succession of don'ts. Negative commands from the outside can break down a child's natural inhibition. The role of the Alexander teacher is essentially that of a facilitator. Teaching becomes a learning situation in which both are students helping each other to experience growth and development.

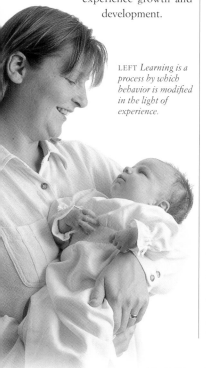

LEFT *Learning is a process by which behavior is modified in the light of experience.*

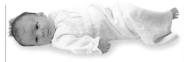

LYING

First Three Months

In the first three months of the baby's life, lack of head control is the important factor in how he moves. He develops the grasping reflex.

At Four Months

At approximately four months, he has head control – he takes pleasure in his own voice, he plays with his hands, he smiles at all faces. He sits upright unsupported with his hands, free to play.

At Seven Months

At seven months, he is sitting up with his back shaped in a single curve. He explores his environment with his eyes and begins to take solid food.

The Following Months

In the following months, he crawls, he learns to come up from squatting to standing, at first holding onto things for support and then unsupported. He often stops halfway in the bending position. He comes up onto his toes. He stands, he walks, he explores, but always with someone close at hand. He becomes quite a sophisticated problem solver by the end of the first year. All humans and animals show a tendency to walk in circles if they are blindfolded, as in the dark of night, in thick fog, or in a dense forest. To walk in a straight direction necessi-

WELL-BALANCED

tates constant correction of deviation with the help of the eyes. The "circling instinct" is very noticeable in young children and young animals, and is most probably linked to the labyrinth of the inner ear, which provides an important part of the information that assists the balance and posture of the body. He experiences pain with teething. He learns to speak and recognize visual symbols. He moves away from his dependence on his carer; he starts to ask "what is that and why?" Children learn by copying. It is very important that parents and teachers provide clear examples for children to copy. They need to be try to be well coordinated and balanced, and show ease of movement. With these conditions present, concentration is possible. If the people around them are disturbed or overtired and tense, children suffer.

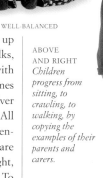

ABOVE AND RIGHT *Children progress from sitting, to crawling, to walking, by copying the examples of their parents and carers.*

UPRIGHT

Discipline and Structure

Do not let your eagerness to help deprive your child of finding out for himself. If you think of learning together, rather than him being the only one who is learning, the whole process could be more creative. Children are eager to find out about everything, but they do need a calm atmosphere and a caring environment in which to learn. They don't respond to being told, but need to know. We need to find ways to arouse and keep their interest and ours alive.

Children are very seldom bored. They do not mind how many times something is repeated. Each time it is new for them; each moment is different. They enjoy sensory stimulation. If, like children, we are happy to be in the moment and not thinking of doing something else, we will not be bored.

There is a growing trend to confuse virtual reality, that is, what we see on film, television, and computer games, with real life. If we passively watch children climbing a tree on a screen, it is not the same experience as climbing a tree. We miss out on sensing the feel of the bark, the movement of our limbs, looking where to put our foot next, the smell and sounds of being up in the leaves, even the real fear of falling. The substitution of television for real life will inevitably impede natural growth and development.

Parents and carers are every child's first teachers. Long before children go to school, parents are guiding them through the early stages of the learning process into the extraordinary world of words, numbers, pictures, and the imagination. The Alexander Technique is concerned with the quality of learning and respects the fact that every individual learns differently. To open up the Alexander Technique to children and make them interested to learn, we have to start at the very beginning, and that is with teaching them inhibition or the ability to say "No" before performing even the simplest action. There is a game that is fun to play with children in order to re-establish "No" in a positive way. Ask a child, "Do you know the magic word?" "No," he replies. Children are delighted when you assure them "That's right, 'No' is the magic word. It can be your secret word. You can say it before you do anything. You can say it before you speak. Nobody needs to know that you are doing it. It is a secret that you share with yourself." This opens up for children a new way of thinking about the word "No." For a child, the idea of inhibition and stopping needs to have a

positive element about it. "No" usually means something negative. When children's understanding of "No" changes, they can begin to think about direction.

The Golden Thread

Most children have a fine sense of natural direction. Once they have stopped doing the wrong thing, very often the right thing does itself. For a child, the word "direction" could be described as a "golden thread running all the way from the top of your head to the soles of your feet, like a bright, shining ribbon, that you do not want to squash or crumple."

By preventing children from developing harmful habitual patterns that impede their health and progress during childhood, we could avoid some of the problems that could beset them as adults. We are often tempted to help our children to walk sooner than they are ready. Mechanical baby walkers are a bad idea since they can give the sensation of movement before the child has acquired the necessary muscular development with which to cope. Folding strollers are equally inappropriate as the spine is collapsed and unsupported, thereby restricting the child's breathing mechanism.

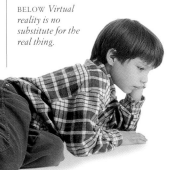
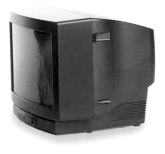

BELOW *Virtual reality is no substitute for the real thing.*

TEACHING THE TECHNIQUE IN SCHOOLS

SUE MERRY

Children start to alter their natural good use when they begin school. When you look at your child working and playing in school or at home, try to observe the whole child. If he is performing an intricate task with his hands, also look at what he is doing with the rest of his body. If your child is collapsed over a drawing or piece of written work, he cannot be coordinating well between hand and eye. If breathing is impaired, he cannot be functioning as well as he might. Feelings of low self-esteem, negativity, and of repeated failure can result.

Our education system is geared toward end-gaining. There are levels of assessment to be achieved, scores to go for, and examinations to be passed. Even kindergarten children are expected to be able to gain certain ends. So although you may be looking for your child to produce good-quality schoolwork, do you have the same interest in what he is doing with his whole self in order to produce such work?

The pressure to master a skill and to produce work that gains approval can be a major contributing factor to deterioration of the use of the self. If you ask your child to try hard to write well, he will simply add more muscle tension to the activity. This is very unhealthy and can very quickly become part of a habitual way of writing, which is difficult to change. It has the opposite of the desired result, producing not better, but more tortuous, handwriting.

> The characteristic note of true happiness is struck when the healthy child is busily engaged in something that interests it.
>
> **F.M. ALEXANDER: *CONSTRUCTIVE CONSCIOUS CONTROL***

Furniture

It is very noticeable how preschool children valiantly attempt to use themselves well – which is their natural use at this age – while attempting to cope with a chair that is far too big and badly designed to allow them to have good use. It is from this uncomfortable situation that we then ask them to perform.

When chairs are too big for children, they are forced to sit with their legs dangling uselessly. You can experience how uncomfortable this is by sitting on a high platform such as the kitchen counter. Sitting like this seems to put a certain amount of strain on the lower back. It is also a very unstable position. If you hold your arms out in front of your body, you will tend to tip forward. Imagine your child in this position with a desk before them. The arms will be used as a support for the body and, as this puts quite a strain on the arms, it is easier to collapse forward onto the table so that the head and upper torso are often also supported by arms on the table. The feet and legs should be supporting the torso, and most very young children strive to get their feet onto the floor at first by sitting on the very edge of the chair. It is natural for most children to seek this connection to the floor through the feet. The natural way of sitting for most young children is in a deep squatting position with both feet beneath the torso and flat on the floor.

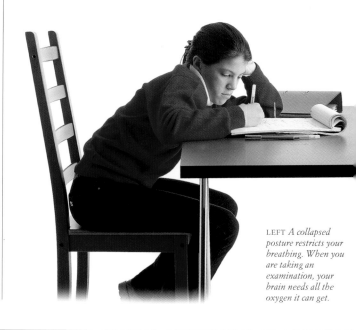

LEFT *A collapsed posture restricts your breathing. When you are taking an examination, your brain needs all the oxygen it can get.*

Children very soon become used to an unnatural way of using themselves when working at a table. They begin to learn bad habits. Such bad use is also habitually associated with whatever activity they undertake while sitting at a table. This is why when children grow and the chairs that they are using are the right size for them, they will usually still sit with their legs dangling uselessly, trailing on the floor, often wrapped around the chair legs. Consequently they will collapse down and use the table in front of them for support. For children to use themselves well while writing, they have to relearn how to write, since writing has become associated with bad use.

Classroom chairs seem to be primarily designed to stack neatly. Usually they are designed with a seat that slopes downward toward the back of the chair. This raises the knees higher than the hips and

BELOW *A dynamic, upright posture facilitates better breathing and more oxygen reaches the brain.*

WRONG FORMULA

Try harder = do more = increase misuse = intensify the conditions that are hampering the achievement of a desired end = be unhappy with the result = try harder = give up = feel you have failed.

What is a child actually learning?
▲ How much muscle tension in the whole body the activity requires.
▲ How to relate to the desk or table before them.
▲ The perspective to view the paper on the desk.
▲ How to sit in the chair provided.

makes it even more difficult for the child to get his feet flat on the floor. The hips tend to slide to the back of the chair. As it is then very difficult to sit upright, the tendency is to slump against the backrest of the chair.

CASE STUDY

Sue Merry
Alexander Technique Teacher, Kingston Primary School

What I often see when a child sits working at a desk is that bad use becomes more difficult to change as time passes. I see children with their feet not flat on the floor, often with their legs contorted. Sometimes their torsos are slumped, and they are often leaning heavily on the table with their arms and even their heads. Their writing arms are usually very tight, probably because they are gripping the pencil. This is largely due to lack of awareness.

I have been working with these problems since 1994. It can be fairly easy through the Alexander Technique to reactivate the good use of infancy using images, games, stories, songs, and a small amount of hands-on work.

It is not an impossible task to teach a child that before he picks up a pencil or crayon, he stops first and checks that he is sitting in a tall way. The child has to understand the feeling of sitting in a tall way with the help of an Alexander teacher. This way every child could be learning a new skill with good use as an inseparable part of that skill. This does not mean not giving praise for good work, but to first give praise for good use. It is also very beneficial for a child to be allowed the time and space to lie semi-supine for a very short time each day.

It is probably much more difficult for adults to adopt this approach to learning, since we have so much more to relearn. With the help of an Alexander teacher, and the understanding and enthusiasm of teachers and parents, it could be possible in primary schools.

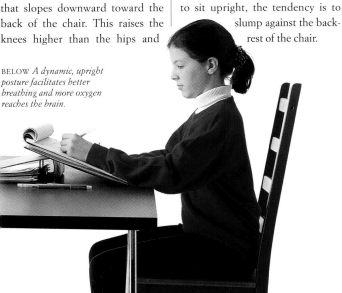

KEEPING
LEARNING ALIVE

Teaching methods are based on the assumption that the student's conception of a new idea is identical to that of the teacher. Students frequently suffer disappointment and failure in their studies because they do not understand what is required of them. Every day in life, misunderstandings occur in trivial as well as very important matters. This process of reasoning is inseparable from what we call "understanding," or "mental conception."

We expect students to acquire knowledge and to be "put right" in matters where they are judged to be "wrong." Parents and carers have their own ideas regarding what the student needs now and in the future and make choices accordingly.

Students are asked to sit up straight, speak out, take a deep

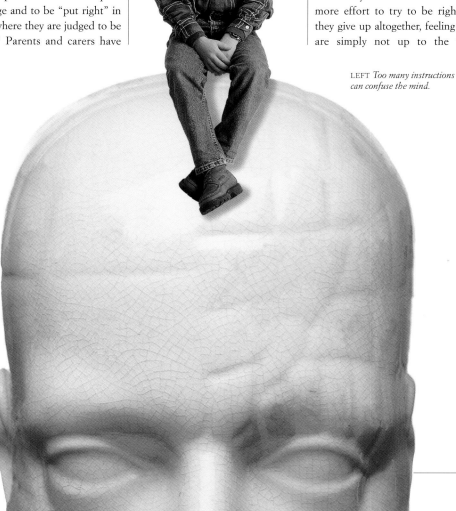

breath, see how quietly they can walk. These are specific end-gaining instructions that rarely include the means whereby the student can carry them out, so they are made to feel it is bad to be wrong, rather than being encouraged to learn from their mistakes. Being wrong makes them fearful which has a very serious effect on breathing. (As Bryon wrote, "Breathless we stand, when feeling most.") Inefficient breathing reducing the amount of oxygen can result in a trance-like condition.

When they become anxious, either they tend to make more and more effort to try to be right, or they give up altogether, feeling they are simply not up to the task.

LEFT *Too many instructions can confuse the mind.*

Self-esteem is lowered with the resultant bad behavior which further complicates the ability to learn.

This sense of hopelessness can make them feel very helpless. Sometimes this causes dramatic outbursts of emotional energy leading to destructive behaviors both to themselves and others. The vicious circle continues until we come to the sad state of labelling some young people "unteachable." Through the Alexander Technique conscious control begins to reduce what Professor Dewey has referred to as our "emotional gusts."

We cannot expect the best results in learning if the student's psychophysical functioning is inadequate. The student's early efforts to learn the curriculum are based on specifics, that is, on "end-gaining" principles of "trying to be right." Long before adolescence is reached, this "end-gaining" procedure will have become established. There will be a reticence and resistant attitude toward accepting new ideas and experiences. There can be a serious deterioration in memory. These defects continue and account for the general lack in many adults to be able to learn and retain information.

Knowledge is of little use in itself; education gives us the ability to link up what we know with our new experiences. The ability to link up ideas is a measure of intelligence and is inseparable from the process of remembering. The value of knowledge lies in our power to associate it with the greater body of information that should have come to us through our years of acquired experience and participation.

Growth and Development of the Adult

The American philosopher and educationalist Professor John Dewey, who died in 1952 at the age of 92, was deeply impressed by the practical benefits and scientific soundness of Alexander's teaching. He said in *Use of the Self*:

Education is the only sure method which mankind possesses for directing its own course. But we have been involved in a vicious circle. Without knowledge of what constitutes a truly normal healthy psychophysical life our professed education is likely to be mis-education.

Education continues throughout life. As we grow older we need not fall into the trap that, as we become less able to do as much as we could, we stop trying. Our life expectancy is much greater today, 75 years as compared with 47 years at the beginning of this century. We can continue to learn new skills and apply the Alexander Technique to how we learn them. Our later years can be educationally enriched.

WRONG WAY TO SOLVE PROBLEMS

Exercise
Teachers and parents mistakenly think that physical exercises, posture training, and breathing exercises will rid children of psychophysical defects. A student's harmful habits acquired during study cannot be remedied by physical exercises.

Specific Correction
Attempts to remedy a specific defect in a badly coordinated student, for instance in handwriting, should take into account the standard of general psychophysical functioning in the student; otherwise, new faults will develop and old ones will be reinforced.

Performance Skills in the Arts

PERFORMERS *in the arts have always valued the Alexander Technique as a way of avoiding tension and finding inspiration. Their bodies are their instruments and have to be finely tuned for them to be able to give artistic expression to their work. They need to play their own true note. Alexander was a Shakespearean actor and today the wheel has come full circle to the Shakespeare's Globe in London. I work at the Globe, as Master of Movement, with the actors, directors, musicians, and teachers. Hamlet's advice holds good for us today, "The purpose of playing ... was, and is, to hold, as twere, the mirror up to nature."*

ABOVE *Do not try too hard. Return to stillness and allow things to happen.*

Performance of any kind demands a high level of energy and coordination. In the mastery of their art, performing artists need directed body use and refined attention to achieve coordination. Alexander Technique helps to develop a very high level of sensitivity and awareness in performers. Then they can begin to discover and discard unwanted postural, movement, and vocal habits that interfere with their art.

Scientific research is confirming that efficiency of breathing and movement, as well as vocal coordination, depend to a large extent on the ease and energy of the upright posture. Being unaware of this results in self-limitation, not just in physiological functioning, but in achieving full potential as a creative, intelligent human being. The Alexander Technique believes there is a connection between full physiological stature and full stature as a creative artist. The human instrument is the only instrument which cannot be tuned by someone else. We can get help from a teacher, but in the end we are the instrument, the player, the tuner, the artistic piece itself, and also the listener.

In this section, the word "posture" will be used. Posture can have the connotation of being static, not dynamic. The term "dynamic posture" suggests a readiness to act. Children, athletes, laborers, artists, and dancers apply to their special activities some phases of dynamic posture they have discovered for themselves or been taught by their instructors or coaches.

Good dynamic posture means using your body in the simplest and most effective way, utilizing muscle contraction and relaxation, balance, coordination, rhythm, and timing, as well as gravity. The smooth integration of all these elements of good dynamic posture will ultimately result in neuro-musculoskeletal performance that is easy, graceful, satisfying, and effective.

PERFORMANCE STRATEGY

Inhibition and direction: Accept that impulses can be counterproductive; stop to establish a readiness, an openness, a willingness to communicate.

The desire to perform: Identify the wish to perform, the character's need or purpose; this will elevate energy levels, increase lengthening and widening; breathe out.

Anticipation: Think about the performance; continue to give preventive directions; "When I go, I will not disturb my alignment any more than necessary."

Go means go: Allow things to happen, accept the unknown, open to the unexpected.

Return to stillness: Inhibit and direct to re-establish full stature; reflect on the performance and ask "Did I stiffen my neck and pull my head back?" "Did I end-gain, did I do too much, did I force my responses, or were they true to the moment and myself?"

ACTING

PENNY CHERNS

An actor has to find a way of locating the differences between himself and the character he is playing. He needs to identify the kind of behavior and life choices the character makes and to discover how these are revealed in the interaction. One of the key tasks of the director is to enable the actor to absorb the character choices.

Preparing for a rehearsal is a vital area; it is necessary to let go of the outside world in order to focus on the task in hand. The Alexander Technique helps to find this new space and centers the actor so he can enter the spirit of the character. The actor's instrument is his body; an instrument has to be tuned so that any note played on it has a clarity and a resonance; the better the quality of the instrument, the richer the note. Language is like music; it has rhythm, energy, and a variety of sound patterns. Every individual uses language differently; the actor has to let it flow through him and his senses so it can resonate and reveal the text. The Technique helps actors to open themselves to this resonance.

When the actor is using his back, he is able to release the breath that gives vocal power as he experiences the moment. He will be neither ahead, behind nor beside himself, but can create from within himself.

Being within yourself also allows for spontaneity; this means that you are not responding on automatic pilot. You are free to respond to the interaction; the ability to receive and then change the energy is the very essence of being in a drama – like in a good ball game. Blocking the other actor's input is like not listening in an argument, considering the alternatives, and having the courage to change your point of view. When improvising, this allows for spontaneity and giving the other actors a chance to contribute their ideas.

Having prepared, the actor can now be in the moment. For the actor there are, however, still hurdles to be crossed before the performance. The first is that moment in rehearsal when he knows his lines and the moves, but having discovered them, and that they work, he is tempted to fix the work. A lot of energy and expression is going on in the facial musculature, but no real energy is flowing between the actors and everybody seems to be operating with the front of the body only. If the actor can be encouraged to let go and trust that the work has fully infiltrated himself, his performance becomes more free. The Alexander Technique allows the actor to be free and in the moment.

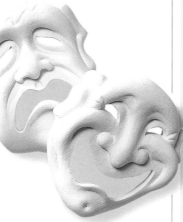

TRAGEDY AND COMEDY

CASE STUDY

Penny Cherns
The London Academy of Music and Dramatic Art

I am a theater and television director, and acting teacher. I came to the Alexander Technique 15 years ago. When I started to have Alexander lessons, the changes in behavior became as apparent to me as the remarkable changes in my body and the improvement in my asthma. I became increasingly aware of more subtle problems in my physical make-up; at the same time I became aware that I was able to prevent (later "inhibit") automatic responses to situations and have a moment of making a choice. It was this concept of making choices that I began to connect more fully to the acting process. I have always been keenly involved in this process, and have been considered an actors' and writers' director and latterly have developed work as an acting teacher. As a director I think it is important to drop the concept of "blocking" the play – a term used colloquially to describe how the actors are moved. The passivity of the image and its fixity are blocks in themselves. Helping the actors to place themselves, to find the dynamic energy of the piece and of their impulses is what the director is really doing.

I have progressively learned more about the acting process over the years because I have been open to understanding it through the connections I have made since I have been studying the Technique. I believe it to be a key method of improving acting and performing, and of immense use to actors in understanding the best ways of using themselves.

DANCING

PERI ASTON

Without movement there is no life. Words applied to the death state include "stiff," "rigid," "cold." However fixed or blocked we appear, there are still thousands of movements going on inside us – flowing, pulsating, breathing, beating. When approaching movement, our problems can be: stiffening, straining, pushing, collapsing, pulling up, pushing down – this blocks energy and stops fluency.

> There is nothing constant in the universe – all ebb and flow and every shape that's born bears in its womb the seed of change.
>
> **OVID: *METAMORPHOSES***

It is so hard to move fluently out of a fixed state – it requires a huge amount of effort. We need to connect with the inner flow which takes us easily into movement.

MOVEMENT

Movement is:
▲ An impulse
▲ A flow of energy – a space to feel the effect of gravity, the body's spring mechanism, a spiral.
▲ A response to a stimulus requiring movement away from or toward expansion or contraction.
▲ A moment of suspense.
▲ Falling in space.
▲ Responding to the contact of the ground.

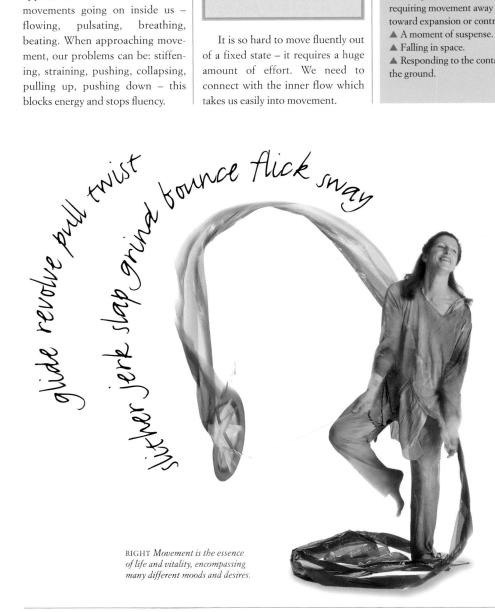

glide revolve pull twist slither jerk slap grind bounce flick sway

RIGHT *Movement is the essence of life and vitality, encompassing many different moods and desires.*

82

The root of the movement is the response to gravity, giving grounded support. Like a tree, the roots form the connections with the earth; the trunk gives flexibility and stability, and the branches are like the arms supported by the roots and trunk. There are three centers of the body from whence you move – the gut, the heart, and the head.

Consider the intention of your movement. When the intention is clear, then the inner thoughts and feelings are conveyed in the movement; there will be clarity, connection, and communication. The moment of preparation to move comes from a still point. The Alexander Technique defines this moment as inhibition. This creates the possibility of choice:

1 To let go of any unnecessary stiffening in the body.

2 To think in which directions you want to go.

3 To connect with the intention.

When you do this, whatever movement you create will have a unity.

> As you from faults would
> pardoned be,
> Let your indulgence set me free.
>
> **WILLIAM SHAKESPEARE:**
> **THE TEMPEST**

There are so many qualities of movement. What unites them is "how" we prepare to move.

Making a quick, strong, pushing movement does not need to be tight, tense, with a lot of effort. It is still a movement of expansion from the center; the head is still freeing forward and upward and the feet letting go into the ground. Conscious control is continual inner exploration, paying attention to what is happening in this moment, not to what you think you want to happen in the next moment. By continuing to say "No," you allow yourself to expand, lengthen, and widen, and you leave yourself open to creative discovery.

ASK THESE QUESTIONS AS YOU MOVE

1. What do I intend by this movement?
2. What do I want to convey?
3. What moves me to move?
4. How does the body want to express it?
5. Where does it want to go?

BELOW *Outer movement is a continuation of inner movement, an impulsive flow of energy.*

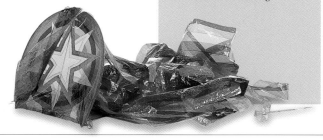

CASE STUDY

Peri Aston
Performance Artist and Alexander Technique Teacher

I always danced, but I was never quite a "dancer." The discipline of ballet forced me into shapes that twisted and contorted my body.

I was never quite a mime. I trained for three years in "mime" at Drama College, but it might more aptly have been called expressive movement. I came to contemporary mime technique late, and never managed to do the three-month/two-year intensive course. I just picked up bits and pieces along the way, struggling to get it right.

I was never quite an actress either. My confidence and voice were ruined at college by attempts to keep my ribs raised while breathing "on the diaphragm." I became afraid to speak.

I started my own creative work again 15 years after leaving college. But I still struggled with my body, pushing it to do things I thought it ought to do. I hung onto the old procedures – hard physical warm-ups, pliés, grands battements, the things I knew. I went on stage tense, and came off in pain, frightened by the clicks in my spine and the strain in my legs.

Then I began my Alexander training and slowly things started to change. First of all, my spine stopped clicking and fixing when I did that certain twisting movement. I prepared for performance by semi-supine and standing thinking. My body was fitter, more supple and flowing, more integrated. I have come full circle, I am dancing again. At age 55, I have become a dancer, but the kind of dancer I want to be, not what I think I ought to be.

MUSIC AND MUSICIANS

Musicians are people who have learned how to listen. Careless rapture does not mean that you do not care, but suggests music played with skill and joy. Creating music should not be stressful, causing you worry and making you overcareful. There is an old Chinese saying that: "The birds of worry and care fly above your head – this you cannot prevent; that they build nests in your hair – this you can stop."

Frank Pierce Jones, in his article on musicians entitled "Awareness, Freedom and Muscular Control" says:

There are musicians – some say there were more of them in the past – who get as much pleasure from a perfor-mance as they give, who always perform easily and well... There are others, however, with equal talent and training, to whom performance and even practice are exhausting, and whose professional lives are short because they lose the mastery of the skills they have acquired. They put forth more effort involving technical problems than the results warrant, and ultimately discover that they have used up their reserves of energy. If they understood the use of them-selves as well as they understand the use of their instruments, such break-downs would be far less frequent.

Tuning the Orchestra

The orchestra is brought into accord by tuning each individual instrument. The quality of the whole relies on the sum of the parts being played by all. Harmony is achieved in this world of sound by increasing the players' awareness of the music, of themselves, of their instruments, of their colleagues, and of the conductor.

Learning how to Learn

The musician needs to understand how to use the instrument he plays. Too often, attention is paid to tuning his instrument, while the equally important job of "tuning" himself is neglected. Another common mistake that the musician makes is that of diverting his attention from the playing itself so he tries to think of something else to "relax his nerves." Neither of these is satisfac-

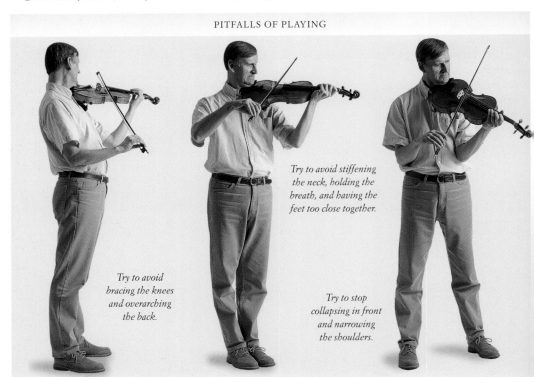

PITFALLS OF PLAYING

Try to avoid stiffening the neck, holding the breath, and having the feet too close together.

Try to avoid bracing the knees and overarching the back.

Try to stop collapsing in front and narrowing the shoulders.

tory and often leads to physical discomfort and tiredness. Things are further complicated if he thinks the piece is difficult – all the old fear responses are generated, and he can end up suffering from pain that can often become debilitating as "nerves" that literally stop his playing. As he begins to employ the primary control, improvements enhance his ability to hold in his mind the complexity of the musical text, the overall shape of the piece, and the sounds he can create. The freedom and release in his back, neck, arms, and fingers provide the possibility of a true rendition of the notes. The miraculous coordination of body, mind, and spirit find their fulfillment in making music.

ANATOMY OF MOVEMENT

The two main masses of muscle, the extensors and flexors, need to be properly stretched out to create the antagonistic pull which maintains the upright structure. The muscles when operating with the opposing pulls create good tone. They are able to act and are ready to act, but do not actually need to do very much. The alternative is to have them both overacting and engaged in a real tug of war. This leads to "pulling down" and stiffness – not recommended for the musician who is trying to play in tune and get the fullest "tone" out of his instrument. When his own muscles are overstretched, the tone can tend to be sharp. When the muscles are flaccid and understretched, the tone can tend to be flat. Appropriate muscle tone allows things to be "in tune."

CASE STUDY

Dorothea Magonet
Royal Academy of Music:
Learning the Alexander Technique
in Music Colleges

Music students spend a great deal of time practicing, rehearsing, auditioning, playing for competitions and performances. They are also under pressure to attain high levels in academic studies.

During regular lessons in the Alexander Technique, students can discover how their habitual and ingrained, ordinary thought processes influence and determine their physical use, and how this can interfere with the acquisition of good technical skills and the desired expressiveness of their music. The student can explore means of stopping this

vicious circle of unconscious and repeated attitudes, postures, and movements.

As the attention becomes more organized and action more coordinated, the student's ability to learn and to take on board new instructions and information is improved. Greater clarity of thought may lead to more concordance between musical intention and technical accomplishment.

The principles of the Alexander Technique provide sound mental skills for the young musician to prevent unnecessary stress and injury; to improve stamina to deal with nervousness before and during performances; to enhance their ability to learn new music; and to make long rehearsals more interesting.

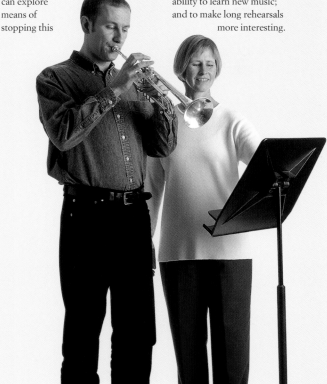

PLAYING STRINGED INSTRUMENTS

FELICITY LIPMAN

Many people think it is necessary to "brace" themselves to stand. In fact, the more we allow our weight to release into the ground, the more the ground will support us and the easier it is to stand. The more we let the ground support us, the less we need to support ourselves.

When we stand with our arms by our sides, the weight is evenly distributed over the soles of the feet. When a violinist plays, his arms are forward and the weight needs to be distributed differently i.e. centered more toward the heels to counterbalance the arms. If this doesn't happen, the violinist may tilt the pelvis, completely altering the relationship of the head, neck, and back and spoiling the integrity of the spine. This restricts breathing and limb movement, and prevents us from releasing body weight into the ground and from receiving the support of the ground.

It is common for a violinist to be unaware that he leans forward or cranes his neck forward or raises his left shoulder in order to reach the violin. These habits completely alter the relationship of the head, neck, and back, causing tension. If we can stand in a natural state of balance ready to receive the violin, then we can play with freedom and poise. We feel freer and lighter when we allow the ground to support our weight. Poise in violin playing comes from a redistribution of weight to accommodate the arms as well as our contact with the ground. This results in a flow of energy, eases the weight of our

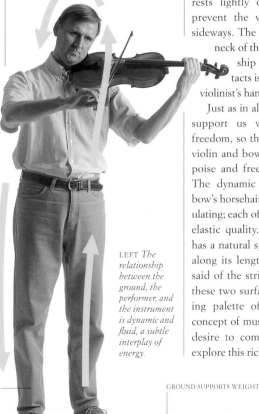

LEFT *The relationship between the ground, the performer, and the instrument is dynamic and fluid, a subtle interplay of energy.*

RELEASED POSTURE ENCOURAGES FLOW OF ENERGY THROUGH THE BODY

GROUND SUPPORTS WEIGHT

shoulders down the back and into the heels, and allows energy to rise up the front of the body.

Violin playing is a much more complex skill than that of standing! However, we can use the same supporting principles. There is a supportive opposition to our weight from the ground – we do not need to push our weight into the ground in order to stand. Similarly, the violin rests on the collarbone, and the head rests lightly on the chin-rest to prevent the violin from slipping sideways. The left hand cradles the neck of the violin. The relationship of each of these contacts is dynamic, as with the violinist's hand on the bow.

Just as in allowing the ground to support us we gain poise and freedom, so the very solidity of the violin and bow allows us this same poise and freedom to play music. The dynamic relationship of the bow's horsehair on the string is stimulating; each of these surfaces has an elastic quality. The horsehair bow has a natural springiness that varies along its length. The same can be said of the string. The interplay of these two surfaces creates a changing palette of colors. Our inner concept of music, together with our desire to communicate it, lets us explore this rich and varied palette.

CASE STUDY

Felicity Lipman

International Performer and
Teacher; Associate of the Royal
Academy of Music; Founder of
the European Suzuki Association

I have experienced many eminent violinists over the years saying what was the "right" or "natural" way to play the violin. Unfortunately, there were major fundamental, physiological differences in understanding, and in the content of their teaching. Why should violinists have a detailed and practical knowledge of physiology? This is not their specialty. Many violinists based their whole teaching on what was appropriate for their individual body, ignoring the fact that there are many different body styles and each bow is unique. In 1992 I resolved to do my Alexander Technique training with Walter Carrington to gain not just a professional knowledge of physiology but a working knowledge – an experience of natural use of the body. Another of my reasons for training as an Alexander Technique teacher was the realization that I lived inside a body I had been taking for granted for decades. Like many musicians I was used to going for my goals with little or no attention to how my body was feeling – the musical idea or thought

was paramount. This realization encouraged me to "inhabit" every nerve fiber in my body. During my training I became aware of tensions and imbalances throughout my body – notably in my neck, my shoulders, particularly the left, and in my pelvis and my legs. I gradually learned how to let go of unnecessary tension by studying a means through which I could release them. I certainly learned all that I had hoped for in my Alexander Technique training – and more! For three years my body had

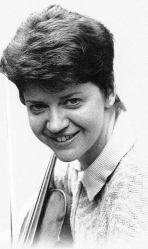

FELICITY LIPMAN

experienced finding what "poise" is. I left the course with a desire to feel at ease and comfortable with any action. I have learned to be aware of tension and to understand the process of releasing it. I have a new sense of balance and of poise, and a freer flow of energy. This has had a profound effect on my violin playing and teaching, which has become less authoritarian. After all, no teacher knows how a pupil's body feels. Teaching violin techniques, I tend to demonstrate the desired actions while the pupil watches not just the individual body part concerned, but how that fits into the whole pattern, e.g. if a child is staring fixedly at my fingers, I ask him to stand back and look at all of me and how the action of the fingers relates to the whole body; then I gently guide the child's limbs in the correct motion and finally ask him to "put it into the computer" i.e. make himself comfortable with the new actions. My teaching language has changed. I tend instinctively not to select words that could indicate forcing or tension but those which keep the whole body free, open, and energized with less about posture than about the feeling of the body in motion. The child absorbs dynamic posture as part of the flow of the movement.

BELOW *The relationship of*
the hand to the instrument is
essential for good playing.

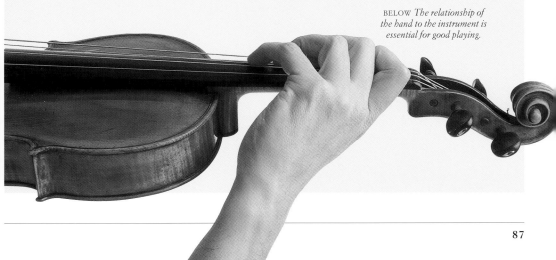

PLAYING KEYBOARD INSTRUMENTS

Understanding and using the instrument well are important considerations in being able to realize your musical skills. The tone of the muscles affects the musical tone that you are producing.

Before you come to play on a keyboard, it helps if you understand some of its geographical detail. You see all these notes that look the same. In fact, they are all different and arranged in a pattern of white notes interspersed with black, raised notes on a large, flat area about four feet long. The music from which you will play is placed above this keyboard. Instead of the score mirroring the keyboard, going from side to side, it is written from top to bottom going from up to down. In order to read the music, your brain has to translate vertical instructions from your eyes into horizontal actions that you perform with your fingers and arms. This takes a great deal of physical practice as you learn the sounds of low and high played on a flat surface.

CASE STUDY

Glen Inanga
Piano Student

I am a postgraduate student at the Royal Academy of Music in London, studying piano. I have had 21 Alexander Technique lessons, which have been invaluable in my development as a musician.

For a long time I had been trying to force the sound out of my instrument and in the process, did harmful things to my body. I am also beginning to learn that the Technique is a lifetime investment, where learning to use the body in the right way minimizes those problems when back pains (for example) begin to crop up.

Lying down on my back for five minutes after a couple of hours of practice helps to heighten the awareness of the relationship between the neck and the back, growing along the spine with the back widening. This helps my body to "breathe" by opening up previously "cramped" positions which come from bad posture, etc.

After an Alexander Technique lesson, my body experiences a certain lightness in feelin, as if it were "uncramped." I feel a unity with the instrument, the seat, the floor below me, and above all with the music.

LEFT *Conscious control ,and released and relaxed awareness allows the musician to express himself fully through his instrument.*

Reading music can often cause you undue anxiety. You tend to peer at the manuscript, narrowing your body and your eyes. This is the exact opposite to what is needed in playing. In order to cover the span of the notes, you need to widen through your back, shoulders, and arms, and feel in your fingers for the sound that you want. All the time you keep a regular pattern of breathing going. When you are faced with a difficult piece of music, one of the first questions to ask yourself is whether you have really understood what is being asked of you. What do these notes tell you about pitch; what do these patterns tell you about rhythm? You need to spend time analyzing and practicing the music in your head before you come to the practical task of playing the notes.

The mechanism of the piano is made up of keys that are mobile. In fact, if you just let your fingers touch the top of the keys, they make no sound at all. The key when touched has its own balanced movement to a certain place where it makes a connection with the hammer that is going to contact the string. When you want to make a sound, you have to put pressure on the key to give it the necessary impetus for this contact. Different qualities of tone – soft, loud, velvet, ringing – need different sorts of pressure. Your mind's ear hears a certain sound which it would like to produce. Over time you will begin to build up a repertoire of sensory appreciation in your eyes, ears, and fingers that allows you to become more skilled at this art of playing.

COLOR STAFF
MARGARET HUBICKI

**PROFESSOR AND EXAMINER
AT THE ROYAL ACADEMY
OF MUSIC, LONDON**

In the early sixties, I invented Color Staff to help two very gifted, eight-year-old string-playing pupils of mine. One, a violinist, easily read the treble clef but not the bass. The other, a cellist, read the bass clef but not the treble. To help them share their knowledge of these clefs, I put together material for their fingers to feel, as well as their eyes, to see the patterns forming the staff.

This material includes a board with five lines printed on it, as well as one with two staves of five lines with a space for middle C. On these boards the different symbols of musical notation can be placed so that the learning of musical theory can be "played with the fingers" in a way that deepens an awareness of what is being studied. A board with the keyboard printed on it is also provided for clarifying and experimenting with the geographical pattern of black and white notes. Small movable pieces are also included – a different color has been used for naming each of the seven alphabetical letters – A, B, C, D, E, F, G – which are the names of the musical sounds. Their use gives the hand and the eye a feeling of their relationship. Treble, bass, and C clefs are provided, as well as small black-and-white symbols, both for pitch and for time. Color Staff does not imply any relationship between sounds and color, but is merely used to link the position of a sound on an instrument to its pitch name and written symbol.

The material provides an experience of the feeling "within information." It is the means whereby detail can be clarified and an awareness created of "what I was talking about" by putting the learner in touch with facts.

BELOW *Color Staff can help to identify the relationship of a musical sound with its place on the clef.*

PATTERNS

Music is essentially composed of patterns – endless different kinds of patterns. The use of Color Staff's separate, different-colored and named pieces is invaluable for identification of these patterns, for example:
1. The relationship – position of a named musical sound with its place on the staff.
2. The repetition of a sound at different pitches.
3. The pattern of scales.
4. Their key signatures.
5. Intervals
6. Chords and their inversions.

I think the idea is excellent… fixing the symbols in the child's imagination as it does. It is useful to have clean staves which, like the blackboard, can be experimented with, and notes put on and off. It is also an excellent way of imprinting the different clefs on the learner's mind.

YEHUDI MENUHIN, K.B.E.

PLAYING WIND INSTRUMENTS

TESS MILLER

Every action, whether opening your instrument case, putting your sheet music on the stand, or playing a phrase on the oboe should be initiated, maintained, and completed with ease and freedom.

Habits with which we play begin with the way we put the oboe together. Therefore it is important to observe yourself as you take out a reed or assemble your oboe. Your thoughts about the forthcoming concert, the difficult musical passages involved, and the fact that you wish you had a better reed will manifest physically, causing you to stiffen and use more tension than necessary.

Before playing, give yourself a moment to check that you have made a connection with your feet on the floor and acknowledge that the ground is supporting you and that you are in balance.

Then give your directions. Ask for your neck to be free so your head can go forward and up... you will then be able to breathe more freely and efficiently, and your body will have at its command all it needs to control the breath and produce the sound that you want to make. It is only when you are out of balance and have lost the connection with the floor that you have to use unnecessary muscular tension.

Similarly, if you are sitting to play, see that the chair is high enough for your thighs to be parallel with the floor (thigh and calf should form a right angle with the knee). Again, acknowledge the contact of your feet with the floor, and of your sitting bones with the chair. The floor is supporting both you and the chair. Never sit on one of those plastic molded chairs with a sloping back seat. Before starting to play, be aware of the natural tidal flow of your breathing. Extend your field of awareness to take in your surroundings. This includes your audience. As you are about to play, see that you bring your oboe to your face and not your face to your oboe.

Check this movement in a mirror. It may feel very strange at first to play without shortening your neck muscles and pulling your head down, and it will probably take a little time to cultivate this new and improved use of yourself. But persevere; the dividends are enormous.

> Gentle breath of yours
> my sails must fill.
>
> **WILLIAM SHAKESPEARE:**
> **THE TEMPEST**

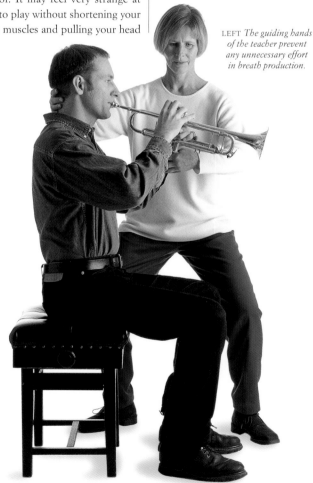

LEFT *The guiding hands of the teacher prevent any unnecessary effort in breath production.*

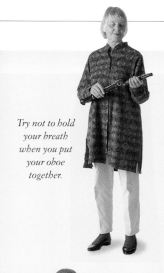

Try not to hold your breath when you put your oboe together.

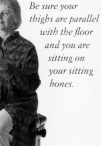

Be sure your thighs are parallel with the floor and you are sitting on your sitting bones.

CASE STUDY

Tess Miller
Alexander Teacher and International Oboist

I have been a professional oboist all my life, playing both as a soloist and in chamber orchestras. Since I was a teenager, I had suffered from a lower back problem. By the time I was in my forties, it was starting to interfere with my work. Sitting for long periods in the orchestra was painful, and I had difficulty carrying my suitcase and instrument on tour. The manager of one of the London chamber orchestras for which I played was herself an Alexander Teacher. She persuaded me to have a trial lesson. I emerged a changed being, with an extraordinary feeling of physical lightness and freedom that persisted for several hours afterward. Regular lessons not only helped my back problem, they also gave me insight into the way I reacted to the stress of my profession. Being a musician makes tough demands on one, both physically and psychologically. Through the Alexander Technique I am discovering how my "use" affects my functioning.

Over the years I had acquired poor habits of the use of myself when playing the oboe (i.e. pulling my head and neck forward and down and tensing my shoulders). This had a knock-on effect on my breath control, my ability to articulate the oboe reed quickly with the tip of my tongue, and also the way I responded to "producing the goods" in a concert or when the red light was on in a recording session. As a musician you have to "get it right now." So there is huge incentive to "end-gain" at all costs. I noticed, even when I was

thinking about making my oboe reeds, that I was holding my breath and bracing my knees back!

The Alexander Technique has opened up a new dimension for me, both in my playing and with my oboe teaching. I have also trained to become an Alexander teacher. By inhibition (a means of quickening my observation) and direction, not only am I more at ease with myself, but there is an enhanced freedom in my sound. I have a wider field of awareness that includes my audience. Hitherto my reaction to an audience was to block it off. I am beginning to learn how to be in response to all that is going on, without reacting in my old habitual pattern, which was all too often driven by anxiety and fears, and which resulted in finding myself physically pulled down and mentally less alert. There are moments when I and the oboe are no longer two separate entities. We are a unified resonating whole, participating with the music and being in communication with the audience. I had had tastes of this expanded state before I encountered the Alexander Technique, but I know that the Technique provides a key, a sure means of entry into this sense of being in the moment, and it is just as true for everyday living as it is for playing a musical instrument.

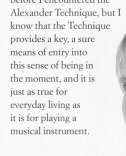

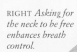

RIGHT *Asking for the neck to be free enhances breath control.*

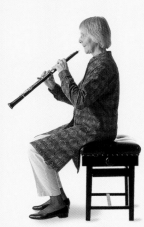

Bring your instrument to your mouth. Do not pull yourself down onto your instrument.

VOICE

ROBERT MACDONALD

Most people are born with an outstanding vocal instrument. Babies make extraordinary sounds, notable for their power, resonance, and emotional variety. We would expect that as we grow in stature and strength the voice would mirror this development. Unfortunately, this is not always the case, and often the aging process brings with it a decline of vocal performance.

When the voice is allowed to operate as a reflex process, it will be free. Once the intention to speak is present, the vocal mechanism is designed to make all the necessary preparations automatically. If we decide to carry out our intention to speak, the body is poised to carry out our intention – the energized

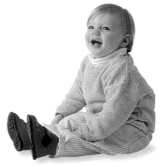

ABOVE *Most babies have excellent natural vocal dexterity.*

breath, the working position of the larynx, the activation of the vocal folds, and the sympathetic activity of the resonators take place in a complex and beautifully coordinated way.

Alexander's perceptions of how he used himself in performance led to the realization that his vocal problem reflected an overall pattern

of misuse, and that overcoming the problem required an evolution of physical and mental awareness. Because the voice is suspended in the body, its free activity depends on the postural mechanisms working efficiently; any inefficiency of the postural body will impose limitations on the voice. The Alexander Technique, by bringing about natural body support, gives the voice the support it needs and the chance to work freely. It then helps us to move into energized activity while avoiding any interference that limits it.

Release of the breathing reflex is fundamental to vocal freedom and resonance. A bell, once struck by an initial attack, will resonate until the sound gradually dies away unless something interferes with the bell, e.g. a hand. Resonance is a process

> Speak the speech, I pray you, as I pronounc'd it to you, trippingly on the tongue, but if you mouth it, as many of our players do, I had as live the town-crier spoke my lines. Nor do not saw the air too much with your hand, thus, but use all gently, for in the very torrent, tempest, and, as I may say, whirlwind of your passion, you must acquire and beget a temperance that may give it smoothness.
>
> **WILLIAM SHAKESPEARE: HAMLET**

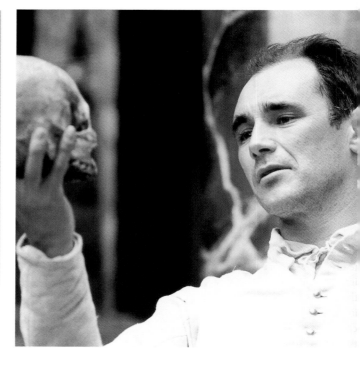

RIGHT *Mark Rylance playing Hamlet at Shakespeare's Globe. Good vocal performance demands full attention to mind, body, and spirit.*

of resounding. The voice works because of an interaction between breath flow, vibration, and the open spaces of the resonators. The role of the voice teacher is to encourage this interactive flow, and to help pupils recognize the role of their upright posture in creating the natural support for this to happen. Postural awareness leads to a greater sense of the gripping and constriction that obstruct the free flow necessary to sound with fullness. Only by realizing our full internal space, and using that to engage the voice, will we be able to communicate and fill a large external space with powerful, resonant, free-flowing sound.

Alexander Technique increases our muscular awareness and helps the performer to make choices about "how" they do what they do. It helps to make the distinction between the essential energy needed for voice and the tensions that limit our vocal potential, leading not only to an increase in power, flexibility, and range, but to an "openness" on every level. Expressing emotion with honesty, clarity, and variety is essential in the vocal arts. In everyday life, the expression of emotion is often accompanied by extreme muscular contraction. Excessive tension in a performer can have the curious effect of blocking the emotion or of making it appear indulgent. The ability to feel the difference between muscular energy and inappropriate tension helps performers to release into emotional expression. It helps them to discard what is unnecessary in performance, and to develop the confidence and simplicity that are the basis of true communication.

RESONANCE

After sound has been made by the action of the breath stream and the vibration of the vocal folds, it can be modified and enhanced by the resonators, giving it audibility and body. It is the inherent size, general shape, and number of apertures (the large ratio of pharyngeal to oral cavity area is a distinguishing feature of the male vocal tract), and the quality and density of the walls of the pharynx, nose, and mouth that will determine the sound frequencies and the unique acoustical patterns that give each voice its distinctive quality.

The resonators can be classed as subglottic, consisting of the thoracic (the lungs, as a large air space, have their own fundamental tone) and tracheal cavities, and supraglottic (consisting of the pharyngeal, oral, and nasal cavities, and the buccal cavities, i.e. the air space between lips, teeth, and cheeks). The subglottic resonators provide air spaces that are set into sympathetic vibration with the vocal folds and act as universal resonators. The principal resonators of the voice are the supraglottic resonators.

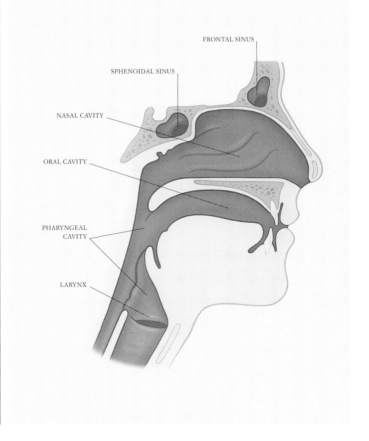

FRONTAL SINUS

SPHENOIDAL SINUS

NASAL CAVITY

ORAL CAVITY

PHARYNGEAL CAVITY

LARYNX

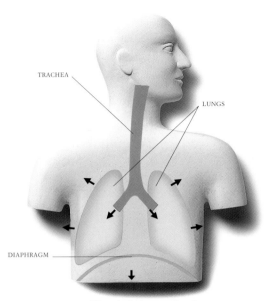

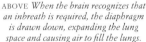

ABOVE *When the brain recognizes that an inbreath is required, the diaphragm is drawn down, expanding the lung space and causing air to fill the lungs.*

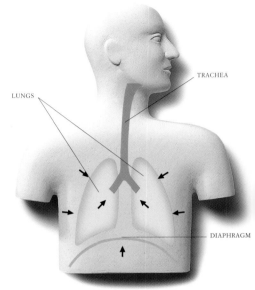

ABOVE *During expiration, the diaphragm relaxes and returns to its customary domed shape, reducing the lung space in preparation for the next inbreath.*

Breathing

The respiratory center of the brain monitors the level of oxygen/carbon dioxide in the lungs. When more breath is required, an impulse is sent to the diaphragm to contract, causing it to flatten and descend. It presses on the abdominal viscera, which drop down and eventually resist the downward movement. The abdomen then acts as a fixed point from which the diaphragm, assisted by the external intercostal muscles, elevates the lower ribs. The lungs, which are attached to the ribcage, are expanded by this movement and the chest is enlarged.

Due to the previous expiration and the subsequent expansion of the lungs by the diaphragm, atmospheric pressure is now greater than lung pressure. That imbalance is quickly adjusted by an automatic, reflex intake of air. Tensions, such as pulling down, sniffing, and gasping, interfere with an effortless intake of breath.

During inspiration, the action of the diaphragm on the viscera and abdominal muscles causes an increase of intra-abdominal pressure. During expiration, this natural build-up of pressure, together with other elastic forces such as the muscular tendons of the chest wall, the lungs, and the torque of the ribs, can decrease the volume of the thoracic cavity independently of any voluntary muscular contraction. This shifting of pressures is the basis of high-performance breathing, and it is important that students experience, early on, the ease and power of this involuntary, elastic cycle.

During expiration the diaphragm needs to relax and rise fully to its domelike shape in readiness for the next inspiration. It is essential that the full stature of the body is maintained, as any degree of "pulling down" or "collapse" will prevent the full rise of the diaphragm, with a consequent imperfect inspiration when it is next activated.

In normal breathing the length of inspiration and expiration are almost equal. When speaking or singing, the length of expiration exceeds the length of inspiration. Students tend to interfere with their breathing reflex in their desire to extend the length of their outbreath and accelerate the speed of their inbreath. This interference is visible in the tension that they use to hold the body and control the breath.

CASE STUDY

Voice Student
*The London Academy of
Music and Dramatic Art (LAMDA)*

Before I started having Alexander lessons, my muscular tension had a negative impact on the performance, the emotion, everything, on the voice. You know you have these tensions, but I think of them as disconnected from the performance, that you are giving this great performance and there are these tensions, but they are not important, whereas in fact they are affecting everything – the vocal quality, the clarity of thought, and the truthfulness of my emotions.

When I did the speech, I did feel a change about halfway through, and that was linked to a forward-and-up head direction which rooted me more and meant that I felt more with the speech. My voice felt very different, much more solid, rooted and how I wanted it to be… and more elastic as well. I felt more able to just do something if I wanted to do it. What was interesting about doing it in the mirror was that… by objectifying yourself you are less stern on yourself so you allowed yourself, time, like when you watch someone else and say, "Just take your time, don't rush, don't

push yourself." I was able to treat myself with that distance and not push myself. The other thing that I noticed was that through watching myself, I was able to spot when things went into a direction that I didn't want them to go in terms of tensing and pushing and immediately apply conscious inhibition, relocate, and start again, so that on each breath there was a new opportunity, a new starting point, and it didn't feel like the first word of the speech was a roller-coaster you get on; if it is a bumpy ride, tough luck, you got on that seat and you can't change once you are on it.

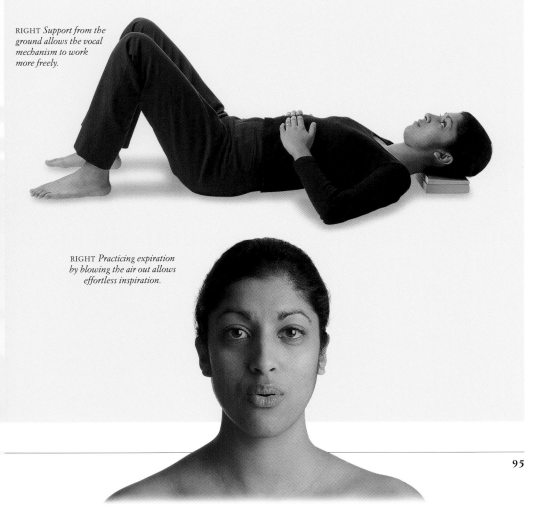

RIGHT *Support from the ground allows the vocal mechanism to work more freely.*

RIGHT *Practicing expiration by blowing the air out allows effortless inspiration.*

Releasing Your Voice

Voice work starts with good breathing. Efficient breathing relies on efficient posture, being able to breathe out and then allow the air into the body without loss of length or width. Bracing up like a soldier or collapsing down like a deflated balloon will disturb natural breathing and interfere with your voice.

Practicing in semi-supine position is good because it helps you to build up the experience of maintaining your full size during vocal exercises. The back in contact with the ground gives support to your body, reducing the tendency to collapse or pull down. The contact with the ground gives you more body feedback, helping you to become aware of unnecessary rigidity or effort, particularly any tendency to retract the head.

Lie in semi-supine (see "Lying Down, Semi-supine," page 60), remembering that this position allows your muscles to release and grow in stature. Any attempt to force or accelerate change will be counterproductive and interfere with your voice (see "End-gaining," page 24). As you lie on the floor with your head supported by the correct height of books, place your hands on your lower ribs. This will allow you to observe the spontaneous changes in your breathing. Now close your mouth and breathe out and in through your nose. If you continue to apply inhibition and direction, air will come in and out through your nose and your breathing will gradually become slower and deeper.

Extend the length of the out-breath so that you slightly increase the amount of breath that you expel from the body. This will stimulate more air to come in. Now when you breathe out, blow the air through your lips. Close your mouth and breathe in through the nose. Repeat the exhalation three times and then stop.

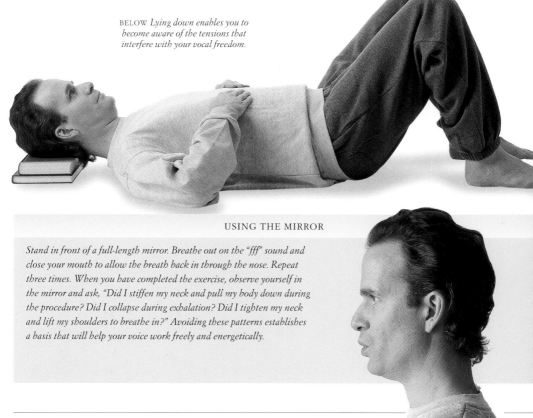

BELOW *Lying down enables you to become aware of the tensions that interfere with your vocal freedom.*

USING THE MIRROR

Stand in front of a full-length mirror. Breathe out on the "fff" sound and close your mouth to allow the breath back in through the nose. Repeat three times. When you have completed the exercise, observe yourself in the mirror and ask, "Did I stiffen my neck and pull my body down during the procedure? Did I collapse during exhalation? Did I tighten my neck and lift my shoulders to breathe in?" Avoiding these patterns establishes a basis that will help your voice work freely and energetically.

At the end of this sequence, it is important that you apply the principles of inhibition and direction, and re-establish full contact with the floor through the nine points of support. As you direct your attention in this way it may help you to answer the question, "In the exercise, did I stiffen my neck and pull my head back?" Being open to this feedback from the body at the end of an exercise is crucial for the growth and development of your voice. It will help you to become aware of the unconscious tensions and muscular patterns that interfere with your voice production. Then you are in a position to avoid them.

In a moment you can try the breathing-out exercise again, but before you do, consider the phrase "conscious involuntary exhalation." Conscious exhalation means that you are aware of the importance of breathing out in order to allow the air back into the body. Lowering the volume of air in the lungs in this way stimulates the breathing reflex. Conscious exhalation also means that you are aware of how important it is to release to your full length through the exercise, and that you place primary importance on maintaining your full free stature through voice exercises.

Involuntary exhalation means that you are allowing the out-breath to happen. It is possible for the movement of the ribcage to take care of itself in response to your simple decision to exhale. Provided that you don't collapse or pull down, the thought to breathe out will generate an easy, powerful, free-flowing out-breath. When emphasis is placed on the direct muscular manipulation of the ribcage, you can become too concerned with trying to achieve the "correct" movement of the rib-cage. Concentrating on maintaining even pressure, or sustaining the breath through a long phrase, can be counterproductive in the early stages of voice work, because it interferes with the inherent ease and spontaneity of the ribs.

When you experience the inherent ease, elasticity, and power of your ribcage, you allow the movement to respond to your decision to breathe out while maintaining your full length. You are giving the movement permission to happen, rather than controlling it.

Now try the exercise again. As you allow yourself to maintain contact with the ground, breathe out on the blowing sound. The formation of the lips provides just the right amount of resistance so that you don't expel the air all at once. This gentle resistance will help to give you the confidence to let your ribs release, and to experience the spontaneous power of the movement.

Shut your lips and allow the air back in through your nose. Repeat this cycle three times. Then stop, give your directions, and gradually re-establish contact with the ground. Mastering this basic exercise will give you a foundation that will improve every aspect of your voice work. Repeat the breathing-out exercise, but on the third exhalation, instead of blowing, hum.

It is the free-flowing breath that eventually becomes sound, and the more you adopt the process of ease and release as opposed to contraction and effort, the more you are establishing the foundation for vocal excellence. Becoming aware of and preventing unnecessary muscular tensions helps you to get the most out of your voice. The time spent at the end of an exercise is crucial because it is taking the necessary time to receive the feedback from the body. By listening to the feedback, we can begin to recognize the difference between energy necessary for vocal expression and when we are creating inappropriate tension.

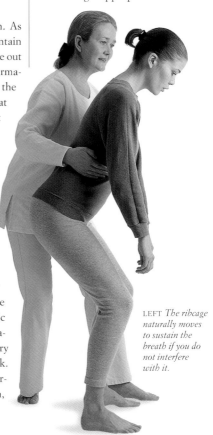

LEFT *The ribcage naturally moves to sustain the breath if you do not interfere with it.*

97

SINGING

Before we developed the art of either oral or written language to communicate with one another, we sang imitatively, echoing the melodies that could be heard in the natural world. These expressions are the deepest feelings of humankind that cut across nationalities, class, and age. They soothe us and stir us up, reduce us to tears and sustain us. "Music hath charms to still the savage beast."

We are designed to make sound. The very word "person" comes from the Latin word *persona*, meaning "that through which sound passes." It refers to the megaphone mask worn by actors in Greco-Roman drama. The Greeks believed that the voice was the soul escaping from the body. The Greek word *psyche*, meaning "soul," has the same root as *psychen*, meaning "to breathe," and the word *pneuma*, meaning "spirit" also means wind.

There is a deep and intimate connection between the breath and the psyche. We could say we truly express ourselves through sound.

EVERYBODY SINGS

When you come to sing, the relevant muscles know what to do. A baby "sings" before she speaks. The first cooing sounds and "Ahs" that you hear are experiments which she makes for hours on end, listening to

Singing is so fine a thing I wish all men would learn to sing.

JOHN CLARE

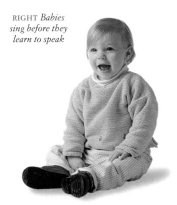

RIGHT *Babies sing before they learn to speak*

There cannot be any sound where there is no movement or percussion of the air. There cannot be any percussion of the air where there is no instrument. There cannot be any instrument without a body.

**LEONARDO DA VINCI,
NOTEBOOKS**

the sounds she can make. Eventually she begins to formulate meaningful sounds and the "Ahs" become "Mama," or a similar sound to which the mother responds. The connection between a sound and a person is forged. The infant has found a way of letting her mother know her needs through sound. We sing first – song lives in the hind brain, the old part in human evolutionary terms.

Singers often fall into the habit of using too much breath to sing. Of course you need breath, but so often the initial intake is miscalculated. A particular relationship between the pressure of breath and the vocal folds is necessary to create a beautiful sound, and the lengthening of the stature creates the overall framework that the voice needs to work well. Overbreathing disrupts that interaction. You will know when you are overbreathing – you stiffen your neck and shorten and narrow your body.

The actual sound of your voice is affected by breath. It is possible to push too much breath through the glottis and give an audibly breathy or even husky quality to the voice. If you do this, you will be wasting air and not be able to sing and sustain long phrases. The exhalation will be more like a sigh that escapes unavoidably. When the quality of breathiness is required in the voice, such as for jazz and blues singing, then there is no problem. But when this vocal quality is not wanted, it causes great distress for singers. They are advised to "get onto their breath," but often lack the ability to know how to do this. The Alexander Technique helps to reduce this habit by connecting the voice and the breath (see pages 64–65).

The tendency to stiffen the legs also causes problems for singers. When this happens, the feet are flattened onto the floor and the "Bubbling Spring," the arch, is tightened. As the legs relate muscularly to the root of the diaphragm, there is a subsequent tightening in this muscle, and this can lead to the production of a restricted sound. Instead of the voice being on the wheel of the breath, it seems to be trapped in the spokes. When the legs and feet are freely connected to the back and diaphragm, the voice can flow out like a fountain.

> When I hear a voice that is not coming out fully, energized and present, then I know there is nothing coming up from the source.
>
> **DAVID CAREY,**
> **SENIOR VOICE LECTURER,**
> **CENTRAL SCHOOL OF SPEECH**
> **AND DRAMA, LONDON**

SUGGESTIONS FOR SINGING PRACTICE

❧ Stop any immediate response to prepare to sing. This can be very difficult because as soon as you hear the accompanist's first notes, you are ready to go for it.

❧ Give the new directions that allow you to stand at your full height by letting your head nod forward in order to go up. Do not look up for guidance; be musically prepared and you will not need help.

❧ Do some whispered "Ahs."

❧ Gently and easily hum with your mouth closed.

❧ Begin to hum and then open your mouth and keep humming so the sound stays inside.

❧ Hum, then open your mouth while still humming, then sing "Ah" as a sustained note.

❧ Begin to sing, but consciously consider how you are singing. Stop if you find yourself going back to your old habits of overpreparing and tightening.

❧ Try not to anticipate problems, and do not allow the high notes to make you frightened and think you need to push.

❧ Enjoy it!

THE SUSPENSORY MECHANISM OF THE LARYNX

The larynx is suspended by a muscular network that stretches it in four different directions. These muscles operate in opposition to each other. The antagonistic stretch brings about the "suspension" of the larynx and makes the proper closure of the vocal folds possible. Unlocking the voice depends on the lengthened stretch of these opposing forces. If the suspensory mechanism is functioning poorly, then it will be difficult to achieve a "low-lying" larynx, and singing will require an effort. It is clear, if we observe the attachment points, that the balance of the head and lengthening and widening in stature are crucial in bringing about the antagonistic stretch. An abundant supply of nerves allow the movement of the larynx to be precisely controlled.

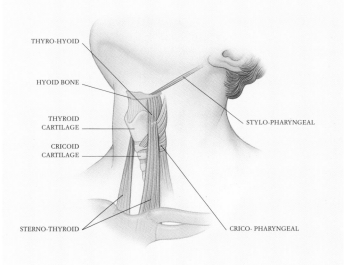

THYRO-HYOID

HYOID BONE

THYROID CARTILAGE

CRICOID CARTILAGE

STYLO-PHARYNGEAL

STERNO-THYROID

CRICO- PHARYNGEAL

ANATOMY AND PHYSIOLOGY OF SINGING

The muscles of breathing, the muscles that suspend the larynx, the muscles that open and close the throat, and the muscles of articulation all attach into the overall framework of the body. For these muscles to function freely and to work together, the body must lengthen in stature, creating an antagonistic pull in the musculature and increasing the opportunity to use energy effectively. Take the example of the steering wheel of your car. When you turn it, are you pulling it or are you pushing it? When you pull it down on one side, you are pushing it up on the other. As with the vocal muscles, it is all one push-pull, constantly adjusting the intercostal muscle tension, the relaxation of the diaphragm, and decreasing volume of the thoracic cavity leading to exhaling air from the lungs. These adjustments then affect the distribution of tension in the larynx.

PUBLIC SPEAKING AND PRESENTATION SKILLS

ANNE FREEMAN

Standing up in front of a group of people and offering something of yourself – talent, skill, expertise – is nerve-racking, however small the group and however experienced the performer. There is no exception to this. Any performer who claims not to feel at least some degree of anxiety is one who does not perform to the best of his or her ability.

Those who have to present information in the course of their work are performers, just like any actor or singer. Usually, in career terms, there is just as much riding on their performance. The business audience, like the theater or opera audience, will generally include competitive peers or aspirants, judgmental superiors or observers, as well as actual or potential customers. The basics of preparation are similar: selection of material; learning; rehearsal. The audience receives a similar sequence of impressions – appearance, voice, and ultimately, the text. There are sometimes even props to deal with, such as the dreaded overhead projector or the latest computerized gadget! So presentation skills can rightly be equated with performance skills, and presentation nerves with stage fright.

In teaching presentation and voice, I find the Alexander Technique central to every aspect of working with a wide variety of students requiring this kind of help, from the most senior in management or the professions to the newest trainee.

The Technique informs the essentials of posture, breath, vocal quality, physical dexterity, and efficient and assured movement, as well as being linked at a deeper and more subtle level to the functioning and accessibility of the personality.

Every performance, like every individual, contains two major elements, the external and the internal – how I seem and how I feel. The Alexander Technique underlies both and unites them.

When the neck is free, the head forward and up, the back long and wide, and the breathing low and efficient, the audience will see a poised stance and easy movement. They will hear an attractive, well-placed voice inspiring confidence. They will be able to relax and take in the words, without worrying about whether the performer is going to cope.

Equally important, the Technique supports the internal element. When the body is correctly used and the voice is agile and well articulated; when we know we can inhibit our immediate panic or excitement responses and so remember our text and deliver it honestly; when we can take the time we need to answer even the most difficult questions appropriately, then we can get out of our own way and make a real connection with the audience. The goal in convincing an audience is for the internal and external selves to become the same. When the mind, body, and voice are saying the same thing, the audience knows that we are telling the truth.

The Alexander Technique cannot affect the message, but it has proved fundamental in developing the quality of the messenger.

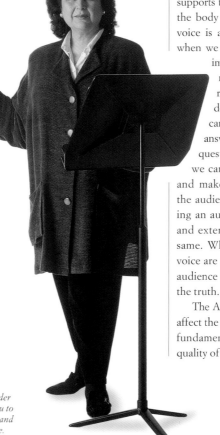

RIGHT *The Alexander Technique allows you to present your subject and yourself with poise.*

Stage fright

We have all experienced the symptoms of stage fright or performance anxiety – sweating, trembling, nausea, and diarrhea. A certain amount of arousal and even anxiety which produces the adrenalin flow can make for a better performance, but too much anxiety can be debilitating. There are a number of factors that can influence the likelihood of how we respond to public performance. Some people are naturally more nervous than others. Some situations are more demanding than others: an important audition or public performance, some pieces of music and dramatic roles, are more difficult than others. If performers are underprepared for an engagement, stage fright always results.

At Shakespeare's Globe Theatre the general level of excitement is increased by the structure of the building. Because it is open to the sky, with 1000 people seated and 500 standing in the yard watching, the actors see the audience and their reactions. This provides a unique

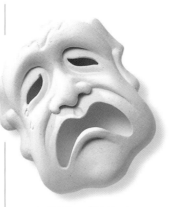

ABOVE *Stage fright involves an increase in muscular tension, which leads to constricted breathing.*

challenge and leads to heightened playing and increased enjoyment.

Alexander organized performances of *Hamlet* and *The Merchant of Venice* at the Old Vic Theatre in London using inexperienced actors. Contrary to expectations, they did not suffer from stage fright even without the services of a prompter. As he explained:

My friends and critics naturally anticipated a wonderful exhibition of "stage fright" on the evening of the first performance, but as a matter of fact not one of my young students had the least apprehension of that terror. By the time they were ready to appear, the idea of "stage fright" was one that seemed to them the merest absurdity. It may be said that they did not understand what was meant by such a condition. And this, although I would not allow a prompter on the nights of the public performances.

F.M. Alexander:
Man's Supreme Inheritance

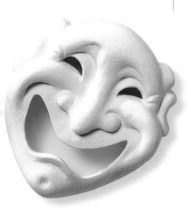

Michelle Kent
Studio Administrator,
Royal College of Music, London

When I commenced lessons in Alexander Technique, I had high expectations of the results I wished to achieve; these have been quickly surpassed.

The most obvious benefit is the feeling of being able to cope and to stand on my own two feet, providing clearer focus in decision-making, greater self-confidence and self-control, leading to a much calmer approach to everything. I have lost the sense of panic I used to get when faced with more than I thought I could cope with. As a result of this new-found security, I feel I am able to provide more support to others.

I have also noticed a marked improvement in my voice, so that I am singing with greater ease (especially high notes, with which I had problems previously). Another consequence is the release of creativity, allowing freedom of thought and opening other channels for relaxation (music, drawing, and writing). Taking part in a jazz music summer school (singing) proved just how valuable these new skills are. New experiences such as this are often daunting and unnerving, but I was able to turn my fast day of dread into a fun and exciting week of learning new skills (vocal improvisation especially) and performing in the club each night without tension in my neck and shoulders.

The increased energy, sense of direction, and inner strength gained have changed my outlook on life dramatically.

PAINTING

ELIZA ANDREWES

The difference between a bad and a good drawing could be said to be the difference between a copy and a personal interpretation of the subject. The Alexander Technique can help the physical activity that leads to the creative activity.

Painting is the equation of:
1. Concept
2. Medium (i.e. the material used)
3. Human body

So often the use of the human body is taken for granted until trouble occurs in the form of pain. Exceptions include Chinese brush-painting and calligraphy, in which body technique is appreciated.

The concept is an intellectual factor, assisted by maximizing the potential of the human body for a particular purpose. When using an easel or painting murals, you have an upright surface at some distance. When doing small paintings, illustrations, or calligraphy, you have a sloping surface close to you.

The medium you use can vary and requires different conditions. If the painting is large-scale, it is often easier to work on the floor. If the paint is very wet, you will need to work on a horizontal surface.

The human body is the implement you use to draw and paint (see Handwriting, page 54). The natural radius of the wrist, elbow, and arm renders the drawing of a perfect circle possible.

DRAWING CIRCLES

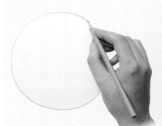

Free wrists allow you to draw moving lines.

If you experience difficulty in drawing free continuous lines, check that you are not holding your breath, stiffening your wrists, and pulling down.

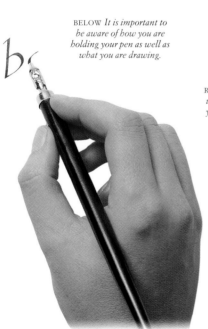

BELOW *It is important to be aware of how you are holding your pen as well as what you are drawing.*

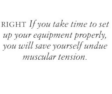

RIGHT *If you take time to set up your equipment properly, you will save yourself undue muscular tension.*

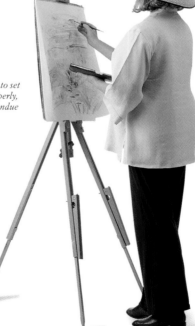

Good Design

When drawing, the line you create follows the circular idea and is curved. In order to make it straight, pressure is needed to push the line upward. As this happens, drawing is no longer a released action, and tension creeps in as concentration increases. This can lead to the habit of holding your breath and hunching your shoulders.

Posture is an important consideration in this skill/art. One of the first decisions is whether to stand or to sit to paint. A second consideration is what distance is required for you to be able to assess your work and get a clear view of the whole.

When sitting, you have the possibility of a close-up focus (e.g. calligraphy, miniature painting, some illustration work). The radius of the whole arm is limited in this position, so the danger of hunching the shoulders and coming down in front needs to be recognized and avoided.

When standing using an easel, you have the possibility of the whole radius of the arm, ideal for releasing the shoulder. The danger in this position is that as you tire, you tend to pull down into the hips. Standing to paint requires a good deal of stamina.

There is a great diversity of equipment available for the painter, but often it is not easily accessible to the beginner outside art school. Necessity is the mother of invention. When you are aware of the height of the work surface you need, you can put a brick at one end of your kitchen table so your drawing board rests on an appropriate slope, or put two crates underneath to raise it to the height of a designer's work table.

Height of table top:
approximately 28 inches/70 cm
from ground. Gradient of slope:
approximately 3½ inches in
12 inches/9 cm in 30 cm.

The Victorian sloping desk was better than the flat tables of today.

Working on the floor on a large surface can be physically demanding, often leading to the bent-back position. Releasing from the hands and knees (crawling) position into painting activity can help. Take breaks to get up and give your directions.

Height of designer's work-top:
36–40 inches/90–100 cm from
ground.

It has an adjustable slope from horizontal to near-vertical with a choice of standing or using a high stool. Like the easel, this is ideal as it allows adjustments to be made easily, and sitting and standing can be alternated. Some pieces of equipment seem to lead to problems. The sketching stool and board can encourage a cramped position and movement. A folding easel and stool chair are more appropriate for sketching.

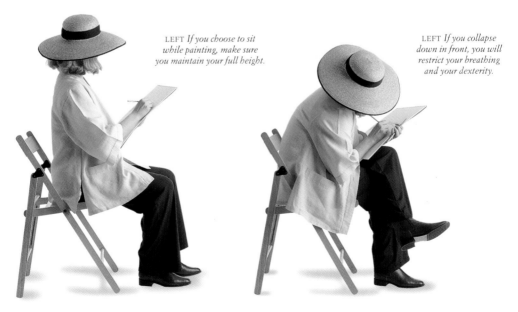

LEFT *If you choose to sit while painting, make sure you maintain your full height.*

LEFT *If you collapse down in front, you will restrict your breathing and your dexterity.*

Sport and Recreation: Conscious Exercise

THE PRACTICE OF *exercising to build muscle and lose weight is a modern one. For the ancient Greeks, exercise was a vital part of daily life, and it was the responsibility of a good citizen to keep himself in good physical condition. Exercise was not an exclusively physical activity, however, but seen as a way of developing the spiritual side of life, a practice of allowing mind and body to work together in harmonious perfection. Mindless exercise would have had no place in the system.*

Alexander questioned the modern attitude to exercise of trying to "get fit." "Fit for what?" was his question. He was concerned that people were not paying enough attention to how they exercised and were in danger of doing themselves more harm than good. He observed that in exercising their muscles, they were creating a lot of inappropriate tension and lowering their awareness of their body. He believed that this way of exercising could increase physical defects and make people less able to manage their bodies easily and efficiently.

The scientific study of exercise has confirmed that, although a certain amount of exercise helps to keep us healthy, when we over-exercise we may be suppressing rather than enhancing the immune system. The idea of achieving peak performance by exercising the body into exhaustion and then letting it recover is being questioned by both sports experts and scientists. It is not just a matter of how much you do, but how efficiently you work. This means that you learn to pay attention to "how" you exercise.

> What (he lacked) was a conscious and proper recognition of the right uses of the parts of his muscular mechanism, since while he uses such parts wrongly, the performance of physical exercises will only increase the defects... while his own consciousness of the act performed and the means and uses of his muscular mechanism will remain unaltered. Therefore before he attempts any form of physical development he must discover... what his defects are...
>
> **F.M. ALEXANDER:**
> ***MAN'S SUPREME INHERITANCE***

Perhaps you have experienced occasions when the harder you tried, the less you achieved. Conscious exercise encourages you to cultivate effortlessness.

Learning to exercise consciously involves paying attention to the signals from your body. How you use your body and how you breathe are the two primary indicators, giving you the feedback that will help you to know the amount of exercise that helps you to reduce stress and the amount that could lead to you over-exercising and actually creating stress.

Although exercise leads to increased activity in your muscles, conscious exercise encourages you to maintain good use throughout dynamic activity. As soon as you find yourself unable to maintain your directions in the activity, your body is telling you that you are exceeding its capacity for easy dynamism and you should stop.

The second indicator is the effectiveness of your breathing. It is often thought acceptable to stretch the body to its maximum

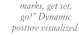

ABOVE *"On your marks, get set, go!" Dynamic posture visualized.*

capacity. By doing this you could end up gasping the air in through the mouth. An alternative perspective on proper exercise asks how active you can be without having to resort to mouth breathing.

Fit for Life

Gradually you will find that you can exert more energy while continuing to maintain good use and efficient breathing. You can then go into a light run, provided that you remain open to the feedback from your self and are prepared to stop and recover when you begin to exceed your body's present capacity. After a while you will find that you start to become mindful of these principles in your day-to-day activities and you will be able to apply them to all your sporting activities.

In competitive events, an athlete is given points for how well the task is performed. In ice skating, ballroom dancing, gymnastics, a top score of ten points may be awarded. High scores come from executing the movement with as few mistakes as possible. The more mistakes, the lower the score. Achieving a high score demands skill and poise, and an understanding of how best to perform the task.

Dynamic posture is posture in motion or in action. Good dynamic posture implies the use of the body or its parts in the simplest and most effective way. For a neuromuscular skeletal performance to be easy, graceful and fulfilling, you need muscle contraction and relaxation, balance, coordination, timing, and rhythm – all working together in complete harmony.

CONSCIOUS EXERCISE

Conscious exercise encourages you to pay attention to:

1. Preparation:
▲ Inhibit and give your directions to achieve your full stature.
▲ Allow the air out and in through the nose.
▲ Be aware of your environment.

2. Start to walk:
▲ Achieve a comfortable speed and rhythm in the body.
▲ Listen to the feedback your body is giving you, and maintain rhythmic nose-breathing.
▲ Increase speed as you continue to be aware of your use and breathing. As soon as you begin to shorten your stature and resort to mouth breathing, then stop and recover:

3. Recovery:
▲ Re-establish your full stature.
▲ Stand still.
▲ Release the shortening muscles and allow yourself to lengthen and widen.
▲ Allow your breathing to recover, ensuring that you are breathing out and in through the nose. Apply these principles to a simple activity before applying them to a sport. Try this experiment while out walking in the park or beside the sea.

CASE STUDY

Frank Trembath
Practitioner of T'ai Chi Chuan and Alexander Teacher

I have been Studying T'ai Chi for 20 years and the Alexander Technique for 15. Both disciplines put forth very similar ideas. During the Alexander lesson the pupil is asked to inhibit the habitual way he uses himself. Before a pupil begins a T'ai Chi Chuan "form" – a series of postures performed in sequence – he is asked to calm himself and empty the mind and "let the head be balanced as if suspended from above." In T'ai Chi we should be neither collapsed nor stiff and rigid, and the muscles should be lengthening. Joints and muscles are never locked or held in fixed positions. The postures are constantly changing and are always in balance. To perform T'ai Chi Chuan correctly, a free neck is absolutely essential. Another important similarity is embodied in the concept of end-gaining. In T'ai Chi Chuan, the importance is not how many forms or movements we have acquired, but the quality of those movements. The Alexander Technique has given me a greater awareness of my musculature, giving me the basis for a better functioning of the muscular skeletal system and reduction of wear and tear.

LEFT *"The Snake Creeps Down."*

RIDING A HORSE

DANIEL PEVSNER, FELLOW OF THE BRITISH HORSE SOCIETY

Humans have ridden horses since the earliest times. The horse has given us both pleasure and service. When we watch riders, we can see a wide range of skills. The harmony between horse and rider can be so great that just a thought from the rider is enough to trigger a response in the horse. The rider has the ability to influence and control the horse through the appropriate use of his own back. This action involves the rider altering the degree of stretch and tension of his spine. He does this very subtly, actually using his back as a working tool that he can activate and adjust at will. When

> Correctly controlled movement of the horse's head and neck – combined with correct use of the rider's body – insures equine equilibrium and efficiency.
>
> **CHARLES HARRIS'S**
> **"THE FUNDAMENTALS OF RIDING –**
> **THEORY AND PRACTICE"**

synchronized with the legs and hands, it has a very powerful influence on the horse. A living body cannot be forced to act in a particular manner, at most it can be coaxed into so doing. This principle, which the Alexander Technique persistently reiterates, is the same for

people and horses. We have the freedom to choose. The Alexander Technique gives guidance.

Comparison between Animal and Human Movement

The horse's head rotates forward and up at a point just behind the ears, called the poll, while the lower jaw softens. This allows breathing and salivation to happen freely. The horse's neck stretches forward, and up with a slight arch, as the back lengthens and widens. The horse's head leads the body. The head direction allows the neck and back to stretch forward and the legs start moving to support the weight. The back is pulsating all the time, and the breathing is regular, giving elasticity and tone to the movement.

WHAT CONSTITUTES A GOOD RIDING POSITION?

A good riding position is often described as "The Classical Seat." The rider should sit upright so that each part of his body rests on that which is immediately below it, so the effect of the weight of the rider reaches the horse in a vertical manner through the seat bones (see page 50). This position offers:

For the rider: security and comfort in the saddle, and the ability to guide the horse with ease and efficiency.

For the horse: reduction in any discomfort that the rider's weight on its back might cause.

This position has to be maintained while the horse is moving simultaneously in the horizontal and vertical directions, curving and moving sideways. This calls for a high degree of firm suppleness in the rider which, can blend and absorb pressure while retaining its resilience and ability to recapture its original shape.

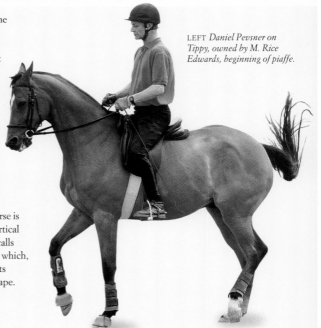

LEFT *Daniel Pevsner on Tippy, owned by M. Rice Edwards, beginning of piaffe.*

ACHIEVING THE CLASSICAL SEAT

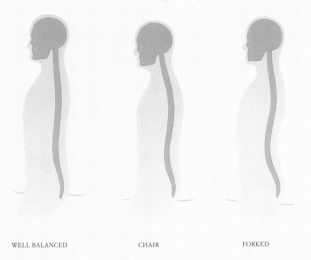

LEFT *Both the skeleton of the horse and the rider need to be able to extend and release in motion.*

The Correct Classical Seat

Compare Alexander Technique seat, spine lengthened, back widened, free working joints, regular breathing, supple body. Weight is supported on the seat bones and the tail bone, which is then cushioned by the buttock muscles.

Chair Seat

Pressure on abdomen, constriction of ribs and diaphragm, reduction of breathing, shoulders raised, chest caved in, upper back rounded, arms stiffened, thighs angled forward.

Forked Seat

Overtense; attempt to achieve "good posture," hollowed back, chest lifted, weight forward, tense hands, legs, head pulled back.

WELL BALANCED   CHAIR   FORKED

Daniel Pevsner
Dressage Instructor, Alexander Teacher, and student of the Spanish Riding School

I began taking Alexander lessons because my back was in pain whenever I got on to a horse, and because I was hoping to improve my riding position. After the first few lessons the pain cleared, and I was changing shape quite dramatically. In time I found a great resemblance between the ideals of good posture and locomotion, as applied to horses or to people. The concepts and the procedures involved in attaining these ideals were not dissimilar. By studying the Technique, I was gaining a better understanding of horsemanship, while my riding experience convinced me of the validity and the soundness of the Technique.

Some months later, the Spanish Riding School of Vienna came to England. The school, regarded as the custodian of the art of horsemanship, has been in existence for over 400 years. The kind of riding practiced in the school is called dressage. At its advanced level, dressage consists of movements which, in equine locomotion, are the equivalent of human dance. What struck me in particular was the superb use and posture of the riders. The riders before me were carrying themselves and acting as if they had all undergone thorough training in the Technique. It then became obvious to me that in order to become a really top-class rider, one would have to develop qualities that would be instantly recognized and appreciated by an Alexander teacher.

RIDING A BICYCLE

JOE SEARBY

When you cycle and everything is going well, the upper body is fairly still, sitting bones contacting the saddle, spine lengthening, head going forward and up. The hands rest gently on the bars. You should be able to lift the hands off the bars without having to sit up much further. If the hands are resting lightly in this way, the elbows can remain free rather than braced and stiff, or sticking out sideways. Contact can be made between the heel of the hand and the handlebars rather than just the fingers. This facilitates release of the hands/wrists onto the bars. An opening out of the shoulders is then encouraged. Handlebars should be wide enough to allow this. The pitched-forward position also puts pressure and strain on the shoulder joints, causing you to raise and round them.

With a better riding position, the lungs are allowed their full expansion and the spine is shock-absorbing. Roads are not always smooth, and shocks through the bike to the lumbar spine are a problem: most cyclists learn early to "lift" themselves out of the saddle over the bumps. Most of the lower-back pain suffered by cyclists is because of the riding position. The only part of the body that should really be moving is the legs. An upright position allows the legs to be used more independently of the torso, a bent-over position encourages the arms and torso to get involved and constricts the hips. The knees need to be brought forward rather than up or down, and away from the ankles and hips.

Move the hips back and down, and calf back and down, and out through the heel. The foot softens onto the pedal, to stop you from pushing with the foot. The ankle needs to be as free as possible. Think of the heel extending back and down to release over the front of the foot. The heels can extend out behind and the toes forward.

Design

The design of the modern bike has the rider's head low down and over the front wheel to cut to a minimum what he presents to the air. This forces the rider to lift his head to see where he is going, encouraging a shortening at the back of the neck. This posture also causes excess bending at the lumbar spine and an extreme forward rotation of the pelvis/hips. It is believed that bending the spine in this way is thought to increase its shock-absorbing abilities! Classic racing advice was to have your saddle nose pointing up anyway. Racing cyclists may suffer temporary loss of fertility, piles and boils during their career.

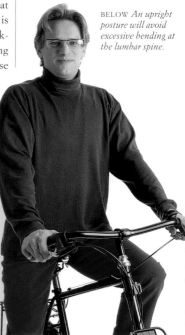

BELOW *An upright posture will avoid excessive bending at the lumbar spine.*

One of the major advantages of making contact between the sitting bones and saddle is that you are better able to influence the direction of the bike through small shifts in body weight. In cycle racing, you corner by leaning into the corner and using the leg as an extra weight, that is, you lean over and stick your knee out, as motorcyclists do in races. If the contact between seat and sitting bones is poor, this ability to move the bike without so much steering is diminished. This becomes important when you are going downhill at 60 mph/100 kph and oversteering could be fatal.

Nevertheless, cyclists tend to suffer few injuries, except through accidents or collisions. The action of cycling is steady and rhythmic, even at high speeds, and a racing cyclist

> ### DAMAGE LIMITATION ADVICE FOR CYCLISTS
>
> ▲ Don't come too far forward in the saddle.
> ▲ Don't tighten your ankles.
> ▲ Don't shorten the back of your neck.
> ▲ Don't bend excessively at the lumbar spine.
> ▲ Don't shorten the hamstrings.
> ▲ Don't hold your breath. in frantic bursts of pedaling.

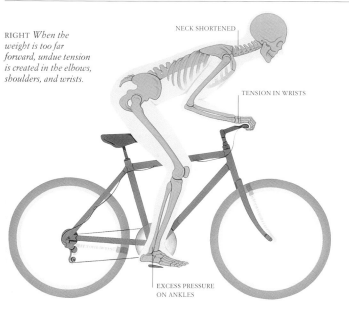

RIGHT *When the weight is too far forward, undue tension is created in the elbows, shoulders, and wrists.*

NECK SHORTENED

TENSION IN WRISTS

EXCESS PRESSURE ON ANKLES

learns how to maintain a steady cadence (rate of pedal stroke) by the use of the gears. By keeping your cadence (for racing cyclists this is something around 100–120 strokes per minute), you avoid large strains on the leg muscles, thus encouraging long muscle with a lot of stamina, rather than short muscle for bursts of activity. Using high gears at low speeds puts huge strains on the legs and very quickly tires them out.

The aim in racing is to convert as much of your energy as possible into forward motion. Therefore the frame and wheels are very stiff with little suspension. Modern mountain bikes often have full suspension front and rear. This is useful if you are going downhill off-road, but on city streets it means your bike is absorbing half your motive energy.

Constant repetition of the pedal-stroke can lead to problems in the long term. A tiny displacement of the foot will be magnified at the

knee joint, and if the knee is then rotated thousands of times with that twist incorporated, you will certainly get knee problems. Shoes that clamp the foot to the pedal are useful as they allow you to use the upstroke of the pedal as well as the downstroke, but the modern clamps require an outward twisting action of the foot that again can lead to knee problems. "Toe-straps" that go over the top of the foot and bind it to the pedal are better. The foot can be drawn straight out and the bindings can be left looser for quick release in case of accident.

Cyclists also suffer from shortening of the hamstrings and of course the muscles of the legs. Most serious cyclists cannot touch their toes. They can also suffer tearing away of the tendons, hernias, and wrist damage (through too much weight being placed on the hands). Many keen cyclists are unaware of the damage they can cause themselves.

Joe Searby
Bicycle Designer and Alexander Technique Teacher

I learned to ride when I was six or seven, but I first started riding a bike every day when I was 11 as a means of getting to school and back. I was lucky enough to be brought up in Cambridge, England, where the bike is common and the hills are rare. After several years of at least six miles a day, I joined the local cycling club and began to train and race regularly. I still ride every day.

Cycling is almost a universal experience. It is both a very common solo and social activity, and a sport. We all want that feeling of freedom and lightness, of effortless motion that freewheeling, with our hands off the handlebars, can give us. But so often we are head-down into the traffic fumes, hell-bent on getting somewhere.

When all directions are going well, cycling is an effortless glide. It is possible to flow along with the muscles of the legs lengthening so that you can't feel the usual effort or tension. The hands on the bars encourage widening of the shoulders and an expansion of the ribcage. It feels as though you are being propelled by an outside energy rather than your own effort. That total combination of awareness and direction rarely lasts long (always another hazard to distract you), but while it does there's nothing like it. That is cycling using the Technique. Without the Alexander Technique, cycling easily becomes a chore, a number of miles to do as fast as possible.

RUNNING

MALCOLM BALK

Good runners run tall, they do not hunch or lean. There is an economy and integrity in their form and movement. They run smoothly. If a runner listens to the whispers, he won't have to listen to the screams. Many times a small niggle, if paid attention to, disappears, and enables a runner to survive and even thrive on the stresses imposed by high-quality training. The problem, if ignored, can turn into something more serious, as many runners and coaches will attest. Repeating something when you are injured or ill often leads to more of the same, or worse. Runners who pound often end up injured. Good runners run lightly – they don't try to dig holes in the ground with each stride. Alexander's belief is that if attention is paid to the means, the ends will take care of themselves. If this belief is taken into the world of training and racing, it allows the runner to take each day as it comes, to have confidence in the process, and to enjoy it more.

RIGHT *The aims of the runner is to be fast, free and light.*

RIGHT *An athlete's track success is based on a relaxed and efficient technique.*

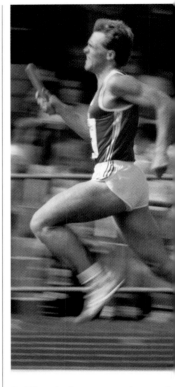

Advice for Runners

❀ Allow your arms to engage the legs through your back. You need to let your shoulders remain free so that the movement of the arms can connect with your legs through the length of the back.

❀ Allow your ankles to release. In order to allow your knees to bend freely, your ankles need to be free. Ask a friend to hold on to your ankle and try to bend your knee. You will find that you have to work hard to overcome the resistance. When they let go, your knee bends much more easily. Any holding in your ankles will make a smooth stride much less likely.

❀ Allow your knees, not your feet, to lead the movement forward. Trying to increase stride length by reaching forward with the foot results in a braking action and slows you down. It can cause you to lean back or sit on your hips rather than running tall.

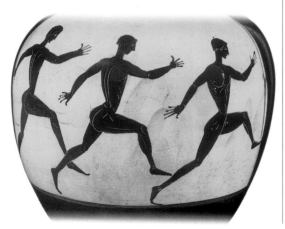

❀ Allow the legs to move in a semi-circular pattern. Good runners allow their legs to turn over in a semi-circular fashion with the heel approaching the buttock at the end of each stride, i.e. the knee bends at least 90 degrees before coming forward. Thinking of your legs moving in a circular way helps you develop a rhythm. This is easier to maintain and modify according to your needs, for example, speeding up or running uphill.

❀ Allow your eyes to look 30–50 yards/30–50 meters ahead. When you look down, you often drop your head and neck as well. This makes you run heavily, as well as putting a strain on your neck and shoulders.

❀ Allow the external direction to be forward and the internal direction to be up. Many runners do not understand that although you may be moving forward in space, your spine does not have to go in the same direction. Ideally, as you are moving forward as a result of the action of your legs and feet, your spine, with your head leading the way, should be lengthening upward. This produces a sensation of lightness in your body, and as a result, your legs do not have to work so hard to move you forward.

❀ Learn to run lightly and quietly. Noisy pounding is a sign that something is wrong. Percy Cerutty suggested you run on the legs, not with the legs. You may be suffering from fatigue, not feeling well, or simply not paying attention. Remember that running lightly has nothing to do with how much you weigh, as anyone with children who like to run around when you are trying to take a nap will attest. It has much more to do with attention – "listening to yourself as you run" – and intention, "thinking up." When runners pound along, they literally jar their whole system. This tendency can be blamed for much of the bad press that running has received in recent years.

❀ Allow your wrists to remain toned, not floppy. Many runners make the mistake of running with their wrists so loose that their hands flop around. They do this because they think they are relaxed, but in fact they are actually creating unnecessary tension in the shoulders.

❀ Allow your arms to move forward and back in a straight line. This is the most effective arm movement to actually propel you forward. A sprinter's upper arm should be parallel to the ground, both when it springs forward and when he pulls it back. You will find that the effort comes in pulling your arm back, not in pushing it forward. You will also realize that pulling your arm back helps your legs pull you forward via your back.

❀ Allow your elbows to remain bent at right angles. A short lever is more efficient since it requires less energy to move. Since you want your arms to contribute to the running action, it is reassuring to know how this can be achieved as effectively and smoothly as possible.

HABITS TO AVOID

▲ Push the body up and let it land heavily on the legs with every stride.
▲ Push with the feet.
▲ Lock the arms onto the trunk or fix the shoulders.
▲ Lock the feet to cross over the midline.
▲ Push (tuck) the pelvis into the legs – it is part of the back.
▲ Allow the head to roll, bob, or wag.
▲ Allow the fists to clench, the wrists to flop, the thumbs to stiffen.
▲ Clench the teeth, tense face, and/or grimace.
▲ Bounce up and down, or roll from side to side.
▲ Push the chest toward the target.
▲ Belly-breathe.

CASE STUDY

Malcolm Balk
Runner and Alexander Technique Teacher

As a competitive athlete I had always run as part of playing baseball and football, and once a year in the high-school track meet. In the late 1970s, I completed five marathons and managed to suffer a wide range of injuries common to many fellow marathoners: Achilles tendonitis, runner's knee, shin splints, calf, quad and hamstring pulls, etc… And although I managed to improve my times, there was a growing concern with a pattern that was becoming more apparent. As I put more and more time, effort and mileage, into running, I was getting less and less return. In 1981, I moved to England to begin training as a teacher of the Alexander Technique. I brought my cello with me and also kept up my running, now focusing on the 800, meters. Although my training included several high sessions on the track familiar to every middle-distance runner, there was a big difference. I was no longer plagued with injuries in spite of maintaining a punishing level of training required for middle-distance running. In my early 40s I maintain a level close to my personal bests. And still, NO INJURIES.

LEFT *As he races, Malcolm Balk exhibits the good use necessary for success.*

SWIMMING

STEVEN SHAW

Swimming is generally regarded as one of the best forms of exercise, promoting a strong sense of health and well-being. The water takes the weight off the vertebrae, allowing for more release of the muscles. However, this is not always the case in practice, as the possibility of misuse is extremely high. Swimming with poor technique can actually do more harm than good. Bad style can aggravate old injuries and cause neck, shoulder, and back pain.

Water can be both frustrating and an extremely liberating medium to move through. When swimming, one finds oneself maneuvering within a substance that is a thousand times denser than air. As you push against it, it seems to do nothing but swirl away from you. On the other hand, the effects of buoyancy balancing the gravitational forces on the body open up a number of new and exciting possibilities for developing greater awareness and freedom of movement.

For a teacher of the Alexander Technique, it is particularly relevant to look at the head-neck-back relationship in swimming. In the buoyant environment of a swimming pool, even small changes in this relationship can have a very considerable effect on the functioning of the body. The common tendency of holding the head out of the water while swimming on the front can produce a significant strain on the whole of the back, which reduces the efficiency of movement. In contrast, releasing the neck so the head rests in the water helps to free the rest of the body, allowing the swimmer to float higher and move with greater ease. Thus, one of the first obstacles to be overcome is the reluctance to place one's face in the water. As a teacher one frequently observes swimmers with their heads held clear of the water who swim relatively fast, but who are thrown into panic when water splashes unexpectedly in their face. Many people often have a false notion that if they submerge their face, they will inevitably breathe in water. Learning to overcome this fear through the application of inhibition is a vital first step. There is little point swimming up and down a pool if you are not completely at ease in water.

The water offers the opportunity to breathe in a much freer way. The physical support provided by the water reduces the requirement for oxygen. Clinical trials have discovered a "diving instinct" that is present in most mammals including human beings; exhaling with the whole face submerged results in a slow-down of the metabolic rate. Tests show significant reductions in both cardiovascular activity and levels of blood pressure. Few swimmers take advantage of these phe-

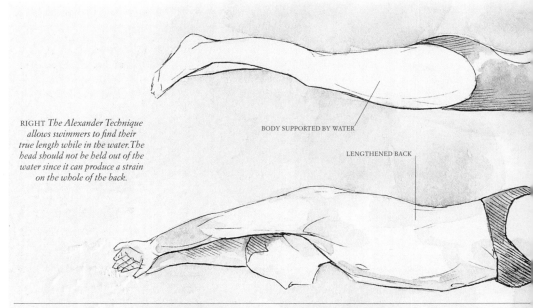

RIGHT *The Alexander Technique allows swimmers to find their true length while in the water. The head should not be held out of the water since it can produce a strain on the whole of the back.*

BODY SUPPORTED BY WATER

LENGTHENED BACK

nomena. While in the water most people are more likely to disturb and interfere with their natural breathing process than they would be outside of the water. This can be attributed partly to the effects of anxiety and partly to an overestimation of the amount of air required to move through the water. People suck in large quantities of air, as if they were about to swim a whole length underwater. If too much air is inhaled, there isn't enough time to exhale it all before the next point of inhalation. This is the major cause of breathlessness and hyperventilation.

In both the crawl and the breaststroke, inhalation ought to be smooth and gentle. Breathing should be focused on the exhalation with the face remaining in the water until all the air is expelled. Then, simply raising the head and opening the mouth allows a natural breathing pattern to provide enough oxygen to continue. Holding the breath underwater confuses and disturbs both the natural breathing mechanism and the rhythm of the stroke.

Stand holding the rail and exhale into the water, first submerging the mouth only, then the mouth and nose, then, finally, the whole of the face. When you feel comfortable and relaxed with the whole of the face under the water, you may let go of the bar and move onto gliding. The amount of time it takes individuals to learn varies tremendously. However, I have yet to meet anyone who, with the right teaching support, has not been able to overcome this fear.

CASE STUDY

Steven Shaw
Author of The Art of Swimming

While training to become an Alexander teacher, I began to notice that I was misusing myself quite badly. Probably the deepest problem I faced concerned my approach to swimming. After years of plowing up and down the pool aiming to increase my speed, I found it difficult to get into the water without working to a set of preset goals such as completing a certain number of lengths in a given time. I realized that my relationship to swimming was one of an extreme end-gainer. As I started to control this tendency, I began to discover that the water offered me a wonderful opportunity to free myself, and for the first time since I was a young child I actually began to enjoy being in the water.

When I began teaching swimming, I found that the tendency toward end-gaining was also a major obstacle for non-competitive swimmers. Many swim in order to get fitter, strengthen their muscles, or lose weight, and have set ideas about what they should do to achieve these aims. Little thought is given to the way they move through the water, and automatic habits take over. It is vital that students reconsider their motivation for being in the water before they can move toward developing a new way of swimming. It is important when learning to improve swimming skills that students do not limit themselves by trying to do it the "right way." What is required is a much more experimental approach. Although pools are public places, feelings of self-consciousness must be overcome in order to develop a new way of being in water.

113

TENNIS
JACK MACDONALD

"You cannot be serious!" How many times has a game of tennis gone from being a lovely invitation to play in the warm sun, with strawberries for tea, to a frenzy of racket-throwing and total disappointment in yourself, the game, and the day? But what is required to avoid this? Concentration is really the major factor in tennis, not just on the score, or whether to play a lob or a volley, but concentration on how you are working yourself. Are you breathing properly? Where is your strength coming from? Are you finding that you stamp across the court while others seem so graceful?

RIGHT *Take your time. Free your neck. Keep your balance. Put your back into it.*

There are times when you have a minute to pause, balance yourself, and then continue with the game. At these points, find the breath again, focus on the space around you, and strive for the key word – fluidity. Often people play whole games of tennis with the words "game, set, match" galloping around their minds and rarely concentrate on each stroke they play. This method of playing an "end" rather than a "game" generally causes us to tense up, which in turn causes us to speed up, which in turn causes us to give up.

The Serve

1. You are at the baseline. If you raise the toes of your front foot, this will guide your weight onto your back foot. At this point, focus on where you want to place the ball and how you are going to do it. Think and breathe out.

2. If you think of the direction above your head as 12 o'clock, it is best to throw the ball above you to about 2 o'clock. This enables you to put your full weight behind you as you jump into the serve.

Stretch and lengthen. Your eyes should be firmly fixed on the ball. Follow the ball with your throwing arm as if reaching for it and at the same time turn your hips as a unit.

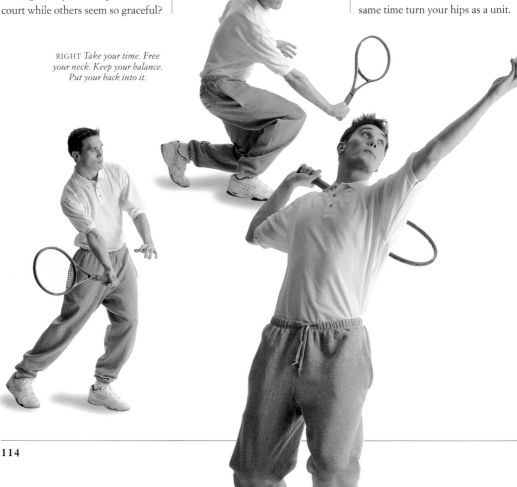

3. So the racket is raised ready for contact with the ball. Your weight should shift onto your forward foot as you make contact. As you keep your body connected, you will be poised for a powerful serve.

4. Try to keep your neck free and your back lengthened and widened. Do not brace your legs or stiffen your ankles. As your throwing arm is dropped, you should simultaneously drop the racket down your back. Now launch toward the moment of contact, while rotating your front hip. Stretch is the buzz word as you use your full size and weight to make contact with the ball.

5. Try to land within the court. Your head should remain up, enabling you to move quickly toward the net, if necessary. Play the game.

HELPFUL TENNIS TIPS

STOP!

1. Use your eyes and expand your vision.

2. Give your directions and come up to your full height.

3. Find your fluidity.

4. Picture the shot you want.

5. Breathe out and find your internal space and your space on court.

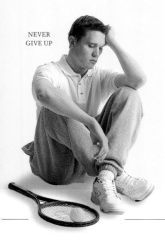

NEVER GIVE UP

CASE STUDY

Jack MacDonald
Tennis Player

I began playing tennis when I was eight years old and found that I had problems in three areas. First, I was growing very fast, but was very skinny. Second, I had a terrible tendency to give up if the going got tough. I felt I had no choice but to be the champion. By not end-gaining or worrying so much about the outcome of the match before I had played a stroke, I began to be able to keep going and not give up. This in turn steadied my nerves, and I did not care so much if I lost a point but just kept playing. Third, I had no control over my breath. This was partly due to being so keen to win I forgot to breathe and also I forgot to have fun, so there was very little laughter on the court. Through stopping and directing, my breathing pattern got easier. By doing whispered "Ahs" I had more breath, and sometimes the thought of something funny released into a laugh which helped enormously. I had more energy and found I could play a five-set match, and even tie-breaks became easier. The Alexander Technique helped me in all these areas and enabled me to give my directions, be aware of lengthening and widening, and use my joints so I knew where my arms and legs started and stopped. This gave me a greater confidence as I realized my space, my posture came together, and my strokes became easier. I feel I can control my height and use it to its full. I gained control over my breath – suddenly my brain and blood were receiving vital oxygen, and my game really picked up.

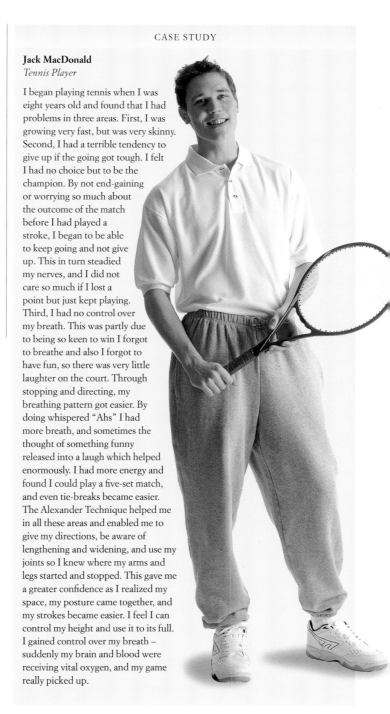

GOLF

GORDON MCCAFFREY

At the time of my first Alexander lesson I had been, for at least 10 years, the stereotypical golf fanatic, and my original motivation for the lessons was simply as an aid to golf improvement. For anyone similarly inclined it may be of interest to read how, through practice of the Technique, golf was transformed for me from an addictive drudgery to an enjoyable sport.

For at one time I was so keen to improve and discover the secret of golf, that I practiced three times weekly and in one frenzied year played and practiced every single day. In looking for this key to perfect golf I supplemented this practice with a comprehensive reading program of golf instructional literature. All the advice of the great players and teachers was analyzed in theory, then attempted on the course – all to no avail. I was left wandering in the literary labyrinth of contradictory instruction where the path of "use all hands" tempted me from the way of "no hands all body," and the direction of good posture was pointed out by guides with clearly distorted spines. It was from this maze that by great luck I stumbled out into the light provided by the Alexander Technique.

RIGHT *Improving your general use of yourself can make your golf game better and increase your enjoyment.*

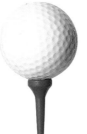

Gordon McCaffrey
*Alexander Teacher
and Amateur Golfer*

It was around 15 years ago I started having lessons in the Alexander Technique and quickly discovered that what the experience did for me overall was much more important than my narrow golfing objective.

In the first six months of lessons, a whole new world of self-observation was opened up to me. Until then I had never given any thought to what I did to myself as I sat in a chair, bent to pick up a book, washed the dishes, etc. My teacher was able to make me aware that my preparation for these acts was wrong and inappropriate. Gradually I began to see clearly that this wrong preparation was present when I played golf, even when I took my clubs out of the locker, teed up my ball, took my grip, or assessed and planned my next shot. So as I gained experience in the prevention of the wrong habitual preparation in my everyday activities, I realized that my golf game was nothing more than a continuation of these activities and not something separate. From then on, my interest in my general use became much more important to me than my previously introverted obsession with golf mechanics.

Amazingly, to me at least, I found that when practicing less and less, I could still play to my low, single-figure handicap. Now, after teaching the Alexander Technique for over ten years, I am certain that my experience with golf, this elimination of practice

RIGHT *Obsessive practice is not the key to perfect golf. Careful self-observation is much more useful.*

and absorption with golf methods, while still playing well, would equally apply to other sports and activities. Of course, the conclusion must not be drawn that an interest in practicing or technique is harmful. It is the use of the self while implementing the instruction or even reading the advice that is all-important. It will soon dawn on any golfer who takes Alexander lessons, as I did, that he or she is involved in something more comprehensive than a golf game.

As my general use improved, so did my golf game, but so also to a far greater extent did my enjoyment of the sport, of being on the course, the stimulation of looking and seeing all around me. This corresponded to a reduction in false concentration causing tension and exhaustion. To be able to enjoy the drive to the course, the game, the company, the drive home, and the rest of the day, is such a happy contrast to my early years in golf. For me, my search for "the secret" was a success, but a far greater secret was revealed along the way.

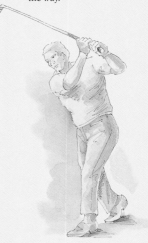

SKIING
VIVIEN GREEN

The Alexander Technique greatly facilitates the learning process for skiing by allowing you to risk things that feel wrong for example the need to lean down the mountain. Wearing skis changes your balance, so practise walking on flat ground first before going on to the slope.

Check that your hips are directly underneath your shoulders and that you are standing in a balanced way, with the weight equally distributed on both feet. Think of the cross-pattern connections – that is, your right hip connecting to your left shoulder and your left hip connecting to your right shoulder as you line up. This will help you to not shorten and contract as you find the body pattern that you need.

Think of widening through your upper back and let your arms hang loosely by your sides. Check that you are not gripping your ski poles.

Gently nod your head forward, and as you do breathe out and let your weight follow the direction of your head. As your weight transfers and moves forward, you can turn the skis and off you go. The conscious awareness that the Alexander Technique teaches you is very important for skiing. This awareness is particularly important when you consider your joints, especially the knee joint and how easily it can be damaged. Because the ankle is immobilized by the boots, greater pressure is exerted on this joint. So getting it well exercised before you go off on the slopes is important. Practice bending and squatting to strengthen your knees and keep them mobile.

Let your knees bend forward so you are leaning onto the front of your ski boots. This is a good moment to check again that you are not over-preparing for your descent by stiffening. Breathe out to release tension.

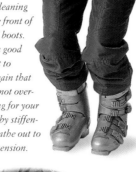

Bend your elbows and hold the poles slightly off the ground. Breathe out again to help release any tension in your shoulders and upper back.

I first started the Alexander Technique when I was pregnant. I used to go along with a huge bump of a baby and after the lesson, because my back had lengthened and widened, there was more space for the baby to move back and the bump had almost disappeared! I decided to try and apply the principles of the Alexander Technique the next time I went skiing. I remember putting on my skis and thinking, keep the neck free, breathe out, lengthen the spine, connect the lower-back muscles, release as I bend my knees. My skiing improved vastly. I floated down the slope, all the time gently reminding myself to smile and breathe out, and the difference was remarkable. When I came to a difficult area, I found myself tensing and losing the fluidity, but with the simple reminder of breathing out and releasing, the whole situation changed.

As with all sports, accidents occur when the fear reflex is activated. The body tenses, and falls become far more serious. So always watch young children and learn to keep their sense of fun and fearlessness, so that when things go awry, the rubber-ball reflex can be activated, laughter comes to the surface, and the tension can be released to make falling an easy art. By the way, never look at adults beginning if you are a beginner – not good examples!

LEFT Be consciously aware of your skiing stance and remind yourself to smile as you descend the slopes.

WORKING OUT

Exercise is very important, but as Alexander pointed out we have to be conscious of "how" we are exercising. We may be consolidating the very patterns of movement that have lowered our level of functioning and fitness in the first place. Before beginning, go through your Alexander directions. Begin with some gentle stretching so that you warm up slowly and consciously. If you rush in to your exercise programmes you stand the good chance of injuring yourself. As in every activity, how you do what you do determines a successful outcome.

Often people make the mistake of stretching in a jerky fashion, or they exert excessive muscular effort to pull themselves into a stretch. Use your body weight as a counter balance to ease you into the stretch. If you listen to your muscles, they will tell you when you have reached

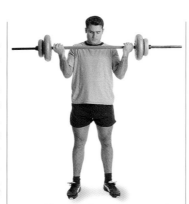

ABOVE *To prevent damage, it is essential to use good technique when working out.*

maximum tension. Stop stretching at this moment and just rest there. Allow your neck to be free so your head can release on the atlanto-occipital joint, drop your shoulders and allow the weight of your arms to help you increase the space through your upper chest. You will find that when you release the resistance in

I see
The lost are like this and their scourge to be
As I am mine, their sweating selves; but worse.

GERARD MANLEY HOPKINS:
CARRION COMFORT

your body, your body weight is then able to do your stretching for you and exert the appropriate "pull" on the muscles.

Rowing Machine

When you sit on the rowing machine, allow your weight to drop down through your sitting bones.

The question of how much effort you should be expending is important, and in the end it is a personal matter. But no matter what your aims are, when using resistance equipment, it is important that you exercise with care and intelligence. If you pull yourself out of shape or generate inappropriate tension in the process, then your results will reflect this. If you avoid tightening in the head-neck-back area, you will sense that you are sitting on a mechanism that glides back and forth, and it will help you to judge when you start to make counter-productive effort. Remember that you are trying to develop strength, but not to the extent of creating shortened muscles that leave the body distorted, out of shape, and muscle bound. So it is important that you register as soon as you start to shorten your stature as you increase muscular energy.

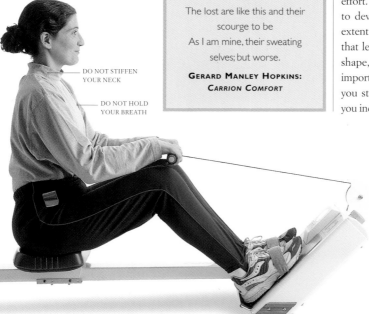

DO NOT STIFFEN YOUR NECK

DO NOT HOLD YOUR BREATH

LEFT *The rowing machine is an excellent piece of resistance equipment that is of great help to the cardiovascular system if used correctly.*

As you start, work with the least resistance possible. This allows you to build up gradually. As you add more resistance, you can be aware of the feedback from your whole body, particularly the head, neck, and upper back, and not just the effort that you are exerting. When you come forward in the machine, it is important that you don't come down in front and restrict the breathing.

Exercise Bike

People on exercise bikes often use inappropriate effort by pulling their heads back, raising their shoulders, and shortening the front of the body. This action distorts the body's framework, and they are failing to exercise the intended muscles.

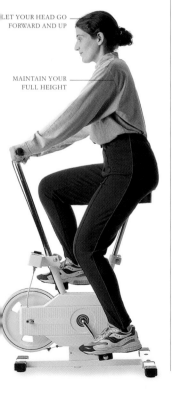

LET YOUR HEAD GO FORWARD AND UP

MAINTAIN YOUR FULL HEIGHT

When you have taken hold of the handles, pause before you start pedaling. Release your neck and let the weight take your arms up and out from your back. Relax up the front of your body. Now let the hips drop down and be aware of the back running up from the pelvis and fanning out into your shoulders and arms. Instead of using just the legs to pedal, think that the legs are an extension of the whole body and that when you lengthen into the action, this allows the whole of your back to share the work.

As you release your muscles and let the legs return to their resting place, allow the air to come in through your nose. Pause for a moment and release the muscles of your neck, back, shoulders, and arms so the full length of the back from the base of your sitting bones to your hands can be restored.

As you get tired, bored, or over-enthusiastic, you may pull your body down indicating that you have reached your limit. Stop the exercise and recover your full height and body integrity before you continue. IF IT HURTS, STOP.

Preparation

The old adage "no gain without pain" has now been proved untrue. Although there may be discomfort as muscles change and develop, this should not be confused with real pain that could cause permanent damage.

There is a growing number of people who train as hard as professional sportsmen while also holding down jobs or careers. Yet they don't have the back-up of physiotherapists, trainers, and doctors and surgeons

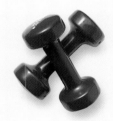

DUMBBELLS

who deal with the injuries of professional sports people. Without that back up, the warning signs of potential injury are often overlooked or missed. People try to work through the pain rather than seeing it as an indication of something wrong. Operations should be a last resort, rather than a way of continuing with the old harmful way of working. The idea of simply enjoying sport is being forgotten. These days it's all about faster times, greater distances, more punishment of the self!

GARDENING

Alexander compared his Technique to gardening, believing that there were no satisfactory short-cuts in either. Gardening, which gives us such pleasure, is also demanding work. Such is our enthusiasm to create our little Eden that we often work for longer and more energetically than is good for us. We get out in April, having not had much exercise over the winter months, and work like mad, ending up putting a fork through our toes or pruning the wrong branch. At the end of the day we are stiff, tired and even injured, with aching muscles, sprained joints, and stretched ligaments. More haste, less speed.

Standing

If we start at ground level, preparing the soil is one of the first jobs we have to do. When using shovels,

forks, and rakes, we need to stand in the upright position. How you take hold of the tool you are using is very important. Quite often, we put too much effort into gripping the handle. See how lightly you can hold the tool without letting it slip from your grasp. So as you begin to rake, dig, and hoe, the amount of energy required will increase, but this does not mean you have to overtighten your grasp. Your long back muscles can do more of the work. Remember to keep your neck free and your head going forward and up as you perform each movement.

This principle applies especially when you are digging; it is not necessary to put huge amounts of energy into the action. Remember that the shovel is designed to cut through the soil and don't dig so hard. When it is laden with soil, remember to counterbalance the heavy weight your arms are carrying by coming back, onto your heels. If you maintain the two-way stretch in your back, you will have more elasticity in your muscles to cope with lifting.

Good advice for gardeners is to take frequent breaks and vary your chores – do not remain too long in any job. When you have done some digging, change to a task that allows you to sit or kneel, or stretch upward.

Sitting and Kneeling

Many jobs in the yard are done in the kneeling position. Edging, weeding, planting in small holes,

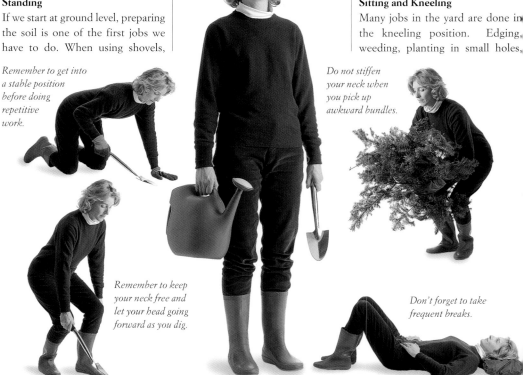

Remember to get into a stable position before doing repetitive work.

Do not stiffen your neck when you pick up awkward bundles.

Remember to keep your neck free and let your head going forward as you dig.

Don't forget to take frequent breaks.

and sowing all take a lot of time – it is no bad thing to be slowed down. The knee joint is not really designed to bear a lot of weight for any length of time. When kneeling is the appropriate position to be in for your task, use a garden mat to help reduce pressure on your knee joints. When you move, crawling on all-fours is an excellent way to move from place to place as you can give your back a rest, allowing it to release and lengthen out in opposite directions (see "Crawling," page 62). Again, do not grasp the clippers or trowel too tightly, and take frequent breaks between jobs.

Bending and Lifting

These essential actions are the most common cause of injuries, often serious. Sacks of soil, bags of refuse, even armfuls of dead leaves need to be moved, but you should be thoughtful about "how" you go about these tasks.

If you feel you have strained your back lifting or carrying, take a few moments to lie in the semi-supine position (see page 60) and allow gravity to help your body return to a released position. Why not look up at the sky and plan what to do next in the yard? Take time to stop and enjoy what your labors are producing.

Pushing and Stretching Up

Pushing a mower or wheelbarrow demands a lot of back muscle work. When you free your neck and allow your back to lengthen and widen, the whole body shares the workload. The dangerous action is often the pulling back of the mower, rather than pushing it. Remember, as in all activities, to breathe out.

When you need to stretch up, you can look up quite freely, but you need to be conscious of how you let your head bend backward. Beware of the tendency to narrow in the upper chest and back. Try not to clutch the tools too tightly.

LEFT AND BELOW *Consciousness of breathing and muscle tension can help you to perform everyday gardening tasks with ease.*

Remember to breathe out when exerting yourself.

Do not overtighten when maneuvering heavy loads. Remember to always stay evenly balanced.

Keep your neck free when you look up.

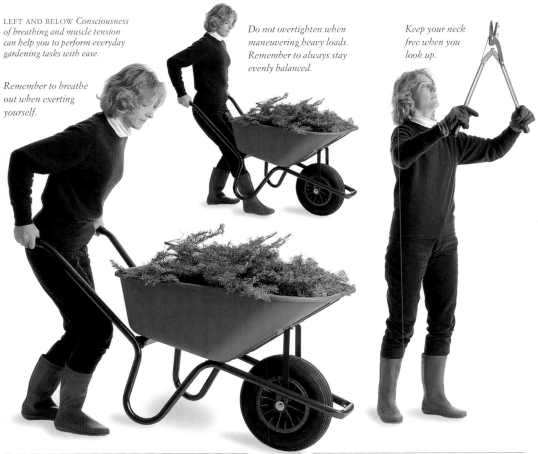

BUILDING AND DECORATING

These days, many of us decide to decorate our own homes. "Do it yourself": the very phrase makes us feel responsible. We do not need an expert, we can do it ourselves. This puts a real responsibility on us. How do we know we can do it? You had better check out "yourself" before assuming you can "do it."

Everyone who has tried to do a job for himself has at some stage blamed the tools – that wretched screwdriver, that hopeless paint-brush that left hairs on every stroke, that useless drill that could not make an impression on the wall. "I'll replace that – it's not worth another moment's grief."

Perhaps we are the problem, not the tools. "A bad workman always blames his tools." Are we bad workmen? And is that "badness" no more than being unconscious of the fact that we are to blame, not the tools? We are the first tool that needs to be checked, long before we abuse the screwdriver, drill or saw.

When you come to painting large surfaces, the usual brush is often replaced by the roller, which spreads a significantly greater area with paint. The danger is that the very nature of a large area full of potentially dripping paint makes the roller quite a tool with which to reckon. The Alexander Technique helps with painting by reminding you to pause before any action. In the case of roller painting, this is essential; otherwise, you end up with an overfilled roller, the need to get it onto the wall and the real fear that it will drip everywhere. These are all stimuli to make you over-tighten and hold your breath, which can lead to stiffness in your shoulders and neck.

BELOW *The Alexander Technique can be used to help you understand how arduous physical work can make your body tense up.*

CASE STUDY

Roger Kidd
Alexander Teacher

Floor tiling is a very physical craft. It involves a lot of lifting and carrying heavy tiles and bags of cement, bending down, kneeling for long periods while reaching and twisting. All these actions have to be carried out carefully with attention to detail, because the end result has to look good.

I was getting aches and stiffness in my lower back and knees. As the jobs had to be done in a reasonable time (for myself and the client), I would then throw myself into the work with more hurried brute strength. This approach made the stiffness worse, but also made me clumsier, forcing me to spend even more time in these awkward positions correcting my mistakes.

The Alexander Technique showed me how I was tensing up well before the point when I could usually feel it (after a long period of kneeling). This then enabled me to avoid these unnecessary tensions before setting about the work, so I could see how I could lift and carry heavy bags of cement without bracing and holding my breath; bend down repeatedly without effort; reach and turn while kneeling without any strain and stiffness. All this let me work more easily and more quickly without the hurry. I am more efficient in my work, and I have more energy because I am no longer wasting it.

MAINTAIN STEADY BREATHING

KEEP BACK LENGTHENED

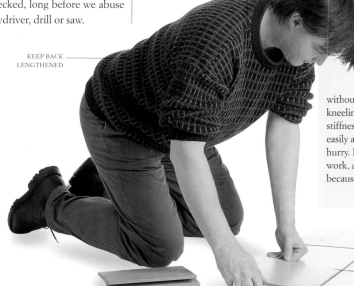

MASSAGE

ANNA PALLANT

Massage, like the Alexander Technique, involves hands-on contact with people. The massage therapist must be constantly aware of the "connectedness of the body" and the integrity of the spine. She must also be able to stop her own tendencies to try too hard to help her patient. Naturally, the aim is to help the person, but by trying too hard the massage therapist can cause unnecessary tension in herself, especially in her shoulders and hands.

If a massage therapist has taken Alexander Technique lessons, her own posture will be comfortable, and she will be able to work with freedom and clarity. Her hands will be light and strong. The direction in which the muscles need to move in order to release will be clearly indicated.

When patients having massage therapy have previously had lessons in the Alexander Technique, they seem to respond very quickly and receive maximum benefits in terms of balance, relaxation, and well-being.

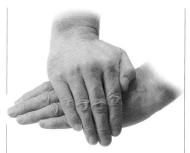

HEALING HANDS

Practical

Working in a position of mechanical advantage is essential when massaging. Massage therapists are standing for most of the day using their arms and hands on their patients. Often their legs can get tired, causing referred pain in the lower back. Applying the principles of the Alexander Technique by remembering to stop and free the neck, to let the head go in a forward-and-up direction, often reduces this tiredness and pain.

MASSAGE TECHNIQUES

Do's
▲ Breathe out while applying pressure through the hands.
▲ Bend in a good way by remembering the position of mechanical advantage.
▲ Widen through the upper back and shoulders.
▲ Think of the shoulders, elbows, and wrists as tunnels.

Don'ts
▲ Hold the breath.
▲ Stiffen the wrists.
▲ Tighten and narrow in the shoulders.
▲ Try too hard to help.

CASE STUDY

Anna Pallant
Artist and Aromatherapist

I have found the Alexander Technique very helpful in my work as an aromatherapist massage practitioner. I started taking Alexander Technique lessons at about the same time as I began my aromatherapy training. At this time I was having frequent headaches and my posture was poor.

Through the Alexander Technique work I learned how my body tenses up, and I learned how to stop and then to direct myself out of these old patterns of use that were causing my problems.

When I see someone in need, I want to be of help to them; but if I try too hard and make too much effort, I often defeat my desired end by becoming tense myself and less effective. So often the more one does, the less productive the massage becomes. It seems the massage is most effective when I am equally conscious of both myself as the massage practitioner and my patient. Then I can be present without being intrusive. Each time I move a limb or work on releasing the spine, I am aware of how their whole system connects up.

One question that my clients often ask at the end of their massage is, "What can I do for myself to help prevent tension, painful back, headache, stiff neck?" My answer would be to have a course of Alexander Technique lessons. It worked for me.

BELOW *The poise, strength, and lightness of the massage therapist will be transmitted to the patient.*

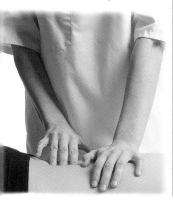

HOUSEHOLD CHORES

We have all benefited from the skills of the designer in our homes. Our kitchens are time-and-motion studies that aim to conserve our energy by reducing how far we have to walk between appliances, by making the height of the work surfaces appropriate, and by generally styling the work surfaces and door handles to be ergonomically correct. Yet despite all these practical advantages, we still manage to spill hot dishes, cut our fingers, slip and fall, and burn the food.

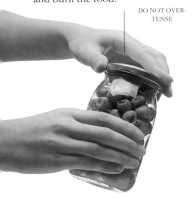

DO NOT OVER-TENSE

A little more study of our own time and motion would pay off. We rush from job to job, without paying due attention to how we are performing. We are always making lists of jobs to be done, from a list of ingredients, to shopping, to the menus, to the order of preparation. What would it be like if we made a few notes for ourselves?

If we had this memo board, we could refer to it as we went from job to job. By taking the time to prepare ourselves before the action, we would be less likely to injure ourselves. Let us look at the familiar job of chopping vegetables.

Chopping

Think of how you are standing before you begin. Do not stiffen your knees or lock your ankles, but allow your knees to flex gently and your hip bones to move slightly back, so you are beginning to bend. When you pick up the knife, try not to grasp it too tightly, and do not hold your breath. When you begin to chop, try not to hunch your shoulders, and try to have your knife sharp, so you do not have to put too much effort into pressing down. When you have chopped for a while, stop and take a break. Move from this position and do some other job for a moment, so your muscles do not lock into the repetitive chopping mode. Taking these momentary breaks will allow you to resume your task efficiently and probably do it faster and better.

Don't put too much effort into simple jobs. Next time you are taking the lid off a jar, check how much you are gripping the jar, and see whether you can unscrew it with half the effort. The same principles apply to any job done in the kitchen. Remember to keep your mind on the job that you have at hand and do not fall into the trap of end-gaining (seeing it finished) or thinking of something else altogether. Each action is complete in itself, so the cup or plate you are washing at this very moment is the only thing that you are thinking about. Thinking about something else to take your mind off what you are doing, because you do not enjoy it, is a pointless exercise. Paying attention to the job at hand makes it interesting.

Lifting and Carrying

Another area that can cause problems is the lifting and carrying of heavy pots and dishes, often full of hot food. Expecting something is going to be heavy to lift often makes you stiffen (see page 48). When you add to this the fear of getting burned, or dropping a carefully and expensively prepared dish on the floor, the excitation of the fear reflex increases and we overtighten.

The way you prepare to lift is very important. Take a moment to free your neck and give your directions, then test the weight of the dish or pot and whether your gloves or oven mitts really protect you from the heat source. So often you only realize that the gloves are not working when you are halfway across the kitchen. Being conscious of how you perform these actions will decrease the likelihood of straining or burning yourself.

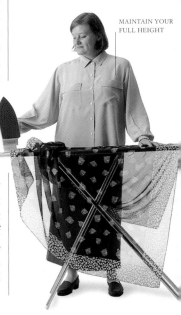

MAINTAIN YOUR FULL HEIGHT

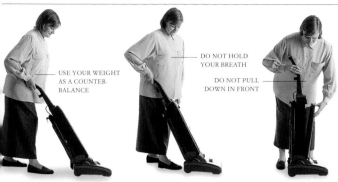

USE YOUR WEIGHT
AS A COUNTER-
BALANCE

DO NOT HOLD
YOUR BREATH

DO NOT PULL
DOWN IN FRONT

LEFT *Be careful when vacuuming that you
let your body weight move forward and
back as a counterbalance to the appliance.*

MEMO BOARD

Remember to:
1. Free your neck.
2. Let your head go forward
and up.
3. Let your back lengthen
and widen.
4. Breathe out.
5. Keep your width in your
upper chest and back.
6. Free your ankles.
7. Free your knees.
8. Think of your shoulders,
elbows, and wrists as tunnels.

Ironing

The way you stand at the ironing board and the very way you get the board set up are important.

Do not grip the iron tightly, nor press down too heavily. If you apply the principles of Inhibition and Direction, you will achieve a good result without finding that you end up with aching shoulders and back.

Vacuuming

Vacuuming is one of the most common sources of back injury in the home. Suddenly, for no apparent reason, our back suddenly gives out, leaving us unable to straighten up or to bend to switch off the power. This may be because we are pushing and pulling a relatively heavy object back and forth, and not paying enough attention to the way we are using our bodies to counterbalance the weight of the appliance. As we continue with the activity, we are lulled into an almost semi-conscious state by the repetitive nature of the physical movement and the numbing sound of the appliance. We are expending physical energy in an almost robotic state. Our muscles decide this is not wise; using too much activity with no thought for how the primary control is working makes them rebel and go into spasm.

How do you stay conscious in a repetitive task? If you keep thinking of your directions and get a good breathing rhythm established, you can avoid the robotic state that can induce muscular reaction that ends in pain or even injury. By waking up the conscious response, even the most seemingly mundane task can be satisfactorily performed.

Sewing

The first thing to do when you want to sew or knit is to consider how you sit. To begin, your weight should be on your sitting bones and your feet on the floor. Your body should not be leaning forward putting weight on the thighs and causing the muscles of the legs and abdomen to lighten. When you pick up your work, you should compensate for the weight of your arms and work by allowing the torso to lean slightly backward in just the same way as a musician has to counterbalance the weight of his instrument. You might find it helpful to try leaning back against a supporting pillow.

The great temptation as you get engrossed in your work is to allow your eyes to draw you nearer and nearer to your work so you end up with the work in your lap and your back a semi-circle.

So support yourself comfortably on a firm pillow, raise your arms toward your eyes, and enjoy your creativity. Whatever one is doing, the important thing is always to remain in balance.

BELOW *When
sewing, be careful
not to let yourself
lean forward as you
become more
engrossed in
the work.*

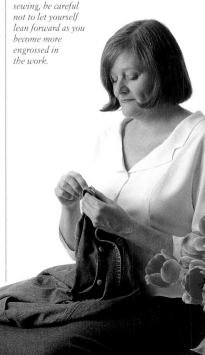

DRIVING A CAR

JOE SEARBY

Regular driving can lead to lower back and disk problems. It is easy to suffer from driving because it is such a demanding task. You are in charge of a potentially lethal instrument, so underlying anxiety levels must be high. You are squashed into a seat, and you have to use both arms and legs almost continually, while also remaining alert and focused.

Most of the problems suffered by drivers (apart from accidents) come from being in a fixed position or posture for long periods while being vibrated and bounced around and hanging onto the steering wheel.

Car seats pose particular problems. The seat slopes backward and in any car more than a few years old is usually too soft and collapsed. It will invariably be more collapsed on one side, usually the right. Many cars offer lumbar supports, but these push the lumbar spine forward, preventing it from flattening and weaken the supporting muscles, exacerbating any present condition. Better is a firm seat wedge that gives more support and encourages a better use of the lower back, allowing it to be mobile and strengthening the postural muscles However, if you are over 5 feet 5 inches, you are unlikely to have the headroom to be able to use a wedge. You could try a triangular-shaped wedge in the corner of the seat where it meets the back, or a piece of wood on the seat is also recommended. People also tend to have the seat back too reclined, so the upper back gets no support at all as they pull themselves forward toward the wheel. Then they have to pull their head back to look forward. Their elbows are rigid, shoulders hunched, head to one side, hands gripping the wheel. Holding the foot over the clutch leads to tension in the whole leg. Allowing the accel-

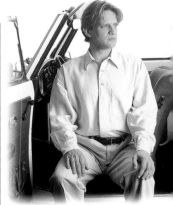

Take your time and breathe out before you set off.

erator foot to fall to one side on long journeys can lead to problems in the knee or ankle.

The angle between the torso and legs is never going to be ideal (always too acute), but you can minimize discomfort by making sure you don't have to stretch for the pedals, also that you are not scrunched up into the steering wheel. Cars are all made for people of average height, so it is bad luck if you're not.

Remember to turn the head freely when looking in the rearview mirror.

Sit well back in the seat, making good contact with the whole of your back.

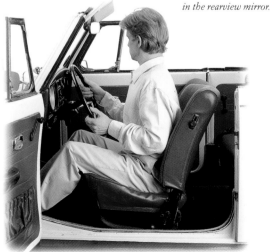

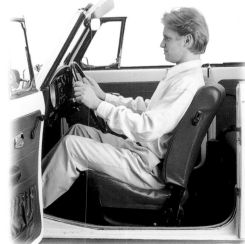

Before you Drive

Take a moment before you get in to the car to stop and stand still. Allow your feet to soften onto the ground. Allow your head to go up to your full height. Let your shoulders release down, away from your ears. Think about the process of driving – about how you are going to get there, not when.

Remember that your state of mind before you set off will be translated into your driving, so if you are anxious or angry or in a rush, take a short time to release these negative emotions. Bring your awareness to your own breathing and allow it to be gentle and easy. Allow the out-breath to carry away any negativity and tension. Avoid anything that has an effect on the central nervous system and increases stress, such as lots of coffee or cigarettes. Get into the car slowly and easily. Stand with your back to the car seat with both feet on the ground. Ease yourself

Let the head turn the whole upper body when you look around.

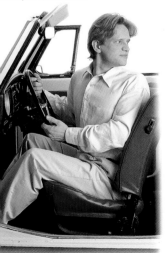

onto the seat and swing both feet into the car. Remember that driving is not automatic – it requires awareness and concentration.

During the Drive

Make sure your left foot does not hover over the clutch, but is resting flat on the floor when not in use. When waiting at lights or junctions, put the car into neutral with the handbrake on. Rest your feet on the floor. It only takes a second to get back into gear again, and you will be less tense when you do so. Occasionally give a slow, gentle push on the steering wheel, using the wrists rather than the whole hand, so that your upper back between the shoulder blades improves its contact with the back of the seat. Pay attention to your elbows. Are they rigid and up in the air? Allow them to be soft and resting easily at your side, pointing down to the floor. Are you gripping the steering wheel too tightly? Relax the fingers and soften the wrists onto the wheel. Imagine you have a glass roof or no roof above your head so you can think about your head going up to the sky. Think about your weight going down into the seat so you are not holding yourself up off the seat. Are your eyes tense? Is your vision fixed on the car in front? Release the eyes by thinking of what you see coming toward you rather than you going toward it. Remember that you have to consider other road users; otherwise, they will have an accident. Does it matter if you let someone in front of you? Does being another 8 feet/3 meters from the front of the line make any difference? How

SITTING POSITION

Sit well back in the seat so that the mid- to upper back makes contact with the seat back. Don't lean your head back on the headrest. Have the back of the seat about 10 degrees behind the vertical so that you are leaning back slightly. Make sure you are not stretching to reach the pedals, but that you are not scrunched up either. Have your hands at the classic ten-to-two on the wheel with the elbows bent so the arms aren't stretched. Allow the wrists rather than the fingers to make the stronger contact with the wheel. Feel that the arms are providing support through the mid-back, making you four-footed. Let your weight down into the seat while allowing your head to go up.

would you wish to be treated by other road users? Treat other drivers accordingly. Don't get caught up in the tension of being late or in a rush. You can't go any faster than the traffic allows, so think about the present moment and how you are driving rather than your eventual destination and how late you are! If you are already late, another few minutes will make no difference. Allow yourself to enjoy the drive. Pay attention to your surroundings outside the car.

After the Drive

Sit for a moment before getting out of the car. Swing around gently in your seat and place both feet on the ground before standing slowly by leading with the head. Stand still, breathe out, and allow your feet to release toward the ground while the head goes up to the sky.

Alexander Technique and Medicine

THE TECHNIQUE IS *primarily educational in nature, but learning and applying it has therapeutic benefits and preventive consequences for the health of the individual. Alexander was certain that the fact that the dynamic relationship of the head and neck facilitates movement of the whole body could be helpful in diagnosing and treating problems. Many doctors who had lessons with him concurred. In 1937, 19 doctors urged in the* British Medical Journal *that the Technique be included in medical training.*

"We are convinced that Alexander is justified in contending that an unsatisfactory manner of use... constitutes a predisposing cause of disorder and disease, and that diagnosis of a patient's troubles must remain incomplete unless the medical man when making the diagnosis takes into consideration the influence of use upon functioning. We deplore the fact that this new field of knowledge and experience, which has been opened up through Alexander's work, has not been investigated by those responsible for the selection of subjects to be studied by medical students." (*British Medical Journal*)

One of the doctors had said earlier that he believed that the Alexander Technique was not another rival to medicine, but an integral and hitherto overlooked factor.

Doctors are skilled in diagnosing disease and prescribing appropriate drugs, or recommending surgical procedures to overcome pain suffered by their patients. Over the last century, they have begun to study the connection between the functioning of the mind and the body. Psychosomatic illness is now recognized as illness induced by the imagination but having no obvious physical symptoms that respond to

testing. The importance for medical science of open-minded observation, of "watching and wondering," is becoming popular again.

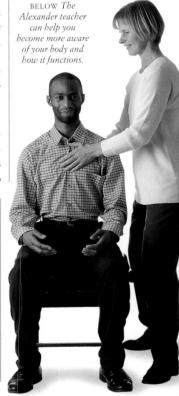

BELOW *The Alexander teacher can help you become more aware of your body and how it functions.*

> Concern is with the sick and convalescent, the aged and crippled. What can be done to prevent the development of physical incapacity and prolong fitness?
>
> **INSTITUTE FOR THE ACHIEVEMENT OF HUMAN POTENTIAL**

> You know that medicines, when well used, restore health to the sick: they will be well used when the doctor, together with his understanding of their nature, shall understand also what man is, what life is, and what constitution and health are.
>
> **LEONARDO DA VINCI, NOTEBOOKS**

PSYCHOSOMATIC ILLNESS

The word psychosomatic has taken on two meanings in modern speech. On one hand, it refers to something phantom, imagined, perhaps made-up, and therefore unreal. In its second sense, it refers to any somatic disorder that is assumed to have at least a partial cognitive or emotional cause. For instance, highly anxious people show a higher incidence of respiratory disorders such as asthma. People in high-pressure, stressful situations show a higher rate of hypertension and gastric dysfunctions. In this sense, the term recognizes that there is a relationship between psychological experience and physiological functioning, that the mind and body interact and have an impact on each other. It appreciates that an illness is no less real because it has a psychological cause. At its most extreme, this position argues that all somatic disorders are, to some degree, rooted in psychological factors.

Alexander teachers are skilled in diagnosing patterns of psychophysical misuse both in themselves and in their students that may limit healthy functioning. They do not diagnose disease, but are looking at disease, the lack of ease that so often leads to malfunctioning.

Learning and practicing the Technique is an exploration of how thought affects muscle activity and how muscle activity affects thought.

In particular, patients with the following conditions will benefit from applying the Technique to the extent that the way they use themselves [their cerebral and neuro-muscular systems] is a factor in the genesis and/or continuance of the particular disorder:

> In nature, there's no blemish
> but the mind.
> None can be called deform'd
> but the unkind.
>
> **WILLIAM SHAKESPEARE:**
> *TWELFTH NIGHT*

▲ Backache or neckache, where posture is a factor
▲ Vocal disorders and vocal cord nodules
▲ Stress
▲ High blood pressure
▲ Asthma
▲ Hyperventilation
▲ Anxiety states (including performance anxiety)
▲ Functional disorders
▲ Osteoarthritis
▲ Temporo mandibular joint syndrome
▲ Scoliosis
▲ Spondylosis
▲ Migraine
▲ Tension headaches
▲ Multiple sclerosis
▲ Parkinson's disease
▲ Rehabilitation after stroke, injury, operation, or other treatment
▲ Dystonias
▲ Nonspecific regional pain syndrome
▲ Cerebral palsy

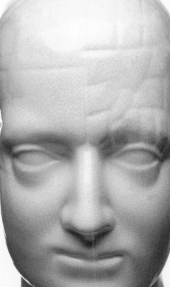

LEFT *Doctors now recognize that psychosomatic illness may have its roots in the patient's emotions and anxieties.*

RESETTING THE HOMEOSTATIC CLOCK

You have inside you a homeostatic clock, whose job is to maintain the normal/natural state of balance in the body – the status quo. All the actions of the homeostatic clock are directed toward a state of affairs where there is no need for any further action. It balances and controls the environment of the body.

A very clear example of the operation of the homeostatic clock is in the ability of the body to maintain a constant temperature. This is a very important part of our healthy survival. Illness is often indicated by "having a temperature," and even an increase of one or two degrees around 98.6°F (37°C) is a sign of an illness and needs to be taken seriously. The opposite is also dangerous, in that if body temperature falls, the condition called hypothermia can develop. This affects cellular activity, and normal body functioning is impaired, often proving fatal for the very young and the elderly. Most of the heat required to maintain constant body temperature is produced by contraction of muscle fibers. Most of the energy is used up in this reaction, but the energy lost as heat helps maintain the constant level of body temperature. On a very simple level, your hands and feet stay warm – a very beneficial side effect of resetting your homeostatic clock. When you work with the Alexander Technique, you bring about certain changes in your body structure. This change also affects your homeostatic clock. The idea of resetting a clock is an appropriate analogy for what happens as you change and reset yourself through the Alexander Technique procedures.

BELOW *Your posture and shape will change through your new way of thinking.*

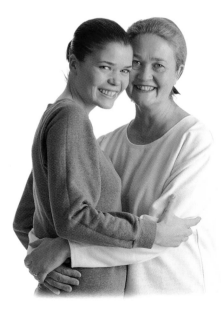

BOBATH CLINIC

Katarina Diss

The following story demonstrates the positive impact of Alexander Technique on cerebral palsy, a disorder of movement and posture due to a defect or lesion of the immature brain which interferes with the motor development.

Whereas in normal child development we progress quite easily from the uncoordinated movements of a newborn baby to the relatively fine coordination of sitting, crawling, standing, walking as well as manipulating, eating, talking, in the child suffering from cerebral palsy this process is interfered with, bringing about abnormal responses to certain stimuli as well as movements inappropriate to the task intended. These problems can range from being wheelchair-bound with severe inability to coordinate the movements of trunk, extremities, head, eye, and mouth, to "minor" problems like walking on tiptoes or the inability to hold a pencil.

When presented with a stimulus, the cerebral palsy patient has very little, if any, choice to respond in any other but the abnormal (pathological) way. The Alexander teacher uses his hands as well as words to help his pupil affected by cerebral palsy to become increasingly aware of the moment in time at which the abnormal movement sets in and how to say "No" to it (inhibit the abnormal response). The teacher aims to show the pupil how to achieve a more normal quality of movement by constructively directing his thoughts.

All this will be a gradual process requiring gentle perseverance over several months/years and no miracle cure. Sometimes it may uncover an associated difficulty that has not been recognized before.

However, as Tony's case study illustrates, it can help to relieve excess tension as well as gradually increase a sense of well-being and ease. There is a good chance of learning something believed impossible before, but above all, it gives the pupil a greater choice by enabling him to say "No" to the unwanted movement.

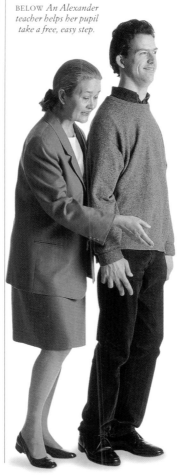

BELOW *An Alexander teacher helps her pupil take a free, easy step.*

MEDICAL REFERRALS

Physicians who are well informed about the Technique are happy to refer their patients to Alexander Technique teachers, and such referrals are on the increase as physicians gain more experience of how cost-effective a course of lessons can be in the management of many disorders.

Lessons are available privately or, in the U.K., can be paid for through the National Health Service either in general practice or in some hospitals like St. Bartholomew's or Westmorland. Health insurance in the United States does not usually cover Alexander Technique, though educated physicians do refer patients

RIGHT *People of all ages can be helped by the Alexander Technique.*

for lessons. Managed health-care companies in the United States are beginning to recognize the value of non-medical approaches to health. Recognition and acceptance are rapidly growing, and the Alexander Technique is available in many institutions, local or state fitness centers, wellness centers, and pain clinics.

A letter in the *British Medical Journal* said:

As practitioners of medicine, we know how great is the need for its (Alexander Technique) resources at the present time, when the strain of existence exacts such a toll even on the healthy. We believe, from practical acquaintance of its effects on ourselves and our patients, that it is adequate to meet that need, if only because it teaches that satisfactory use of the self which is the basis of physical and mental happiness.

Dr. Barlow (1954) demonstrated the re-education procedure with a group of 50 students from the Central School of Speech and Drama in London, England, and reported an improvement for all of them. Speaking as a physician, Dr. Barlow said that he had found the Alexander procedures useful "in such varying conditions as peptic ulcer, spastic colon, ulcerative colitis, eczema, and rheumatoid arthritis" as well as "tension headaches, asthma, low back pain, and fibrositis."

PAIN CONTROL

Pain is mysterious and elusive. In *Hard Times* by Charles Dickens, Mrs. Gradgrind gives an answer that strikes a chord with all of us. When asked:

> *"Are you in pain, dear mother?"* "I think there's a pain somewhere in the room," said Mrs. Gradgrind, "but I couldn't positively say that I have got it."

Dr. Miriam Wohl believes: "It can be a very small difference in functioning that can take someone back over a pain threshold and leave them free of pain. It can make a big difference, especially in the treatment of sciatica." This applies not only to physical pain but in psychological pain – repressed emotions.

Elizabeth Atkinson, Alexander Technique teacher, believes

Emotion is a moving of the feelings. The problem is that people are often reluctant to allow their feelings to move. They get stuck in repetitive situations, limiting their range of movement on a feeling level. We talk a lot about not wanting to limit our range of movement in a physical sense and forget the psychological realm. The Alexander Technique enables you to allow the appropriate movement or deepening of feelings, and so you can begin to experience the difference between more superficial responses, for example, embarrassment, cynicism, flirtatiousness... and deeper, more core responses such as terror, hatred, sexual passion, and joy.

CANCER STUDY

A study of the benefits of Alexander Technique on cancer patients at Mount Vernon Hospital confirmed the following observations:

▲ Patients whose reaction to diagnosis was anger, leading to muscle tension, were helped.

▲ Patients with lung metastases and breathing problems benefited from being in control of breathing.

▲ Patients with a poor prognosis were able to build in a coping mechanism where later lung or skeletal problems are likely.

▲ It is best done before symptoms occur, while patients are still fit enough to travel and learn.

▲ It helped patients to use their waning powers with care, but 100 percent efficiency.

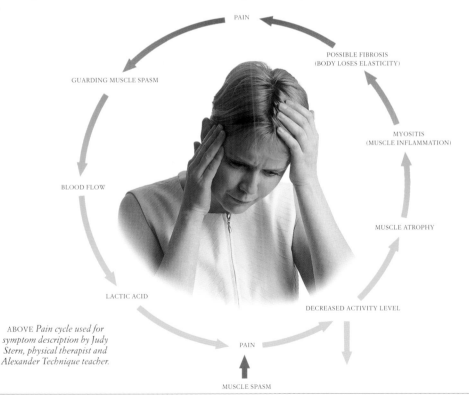

ABOVE *Pain cycle used for symptom description by Judy Stern, physical therapist and Alexander Technique teacher.*

PAIN

POSSIBLE FIBROSIS
(BODY LOSES ELASTICITY)

GUARDING MUSCLE SPASM

MYOSITIS
(MUSCLE INFLAMMATION)

BLOOD FLOW

MUSCLE ATROPHY

LACTIC ACID

DECREASED ACTIVITY LEVEL

PAIN

MUSCLE SPASM

Know Thyself

THE ALEXANDER TECHNIQUE *invites you to take responsibility for yourself, your thoughts, your actions, how you are feeling, and to realize that you have the power to help yourself. It invites you to recognize that the state you are in largely determines how you perceive yourself and the world around you, and that you have the power to change your state. The Technique encourages you to avoid isolating your posture from your thoughts and feelings, but to learn truly to listen to your body. Through improving the awareness of the body, the self is more able to know itself.*

Alexander used the term "sensory appreciation" to refer to the feedback that we get from our bodies. He also used it to refer to the inter-relationships that take place within ourselves: how our thoughts affect our movements and breathing, how our movements affect our feelings, how our emotions can dominate and affect our posture and our capacity for clear thinking. As our sensory appreciation improves, we can become more conscious of how we respond to the constant stimuli from outside and the impulses from inside the self.

> The fault, dear Brutus,
> is not in our stars
> But in ourselves.
>
> **WILLIAM SHAKESPEARE:**
> **JULIUS CAESAR**

FEAR

Humans have always feared the unknown and lived in constant expectation of an attack from their natural enemies. Although we have moved into a civilized state, this old fear remains. We have developed our mental ability, often to the detriment of our physical prowess. Alexander believed that these imbalances should be addressed and that mankind could become alert and ready to deal with the unknown through becoming more conscious.

There is nothing to fear but fear itself – a trite sound-bite that is more than just a clever cover-up. It has a deep meaning within the very make-up of our neurology.

Most of us go through life as if we were in a permanent state of fear.

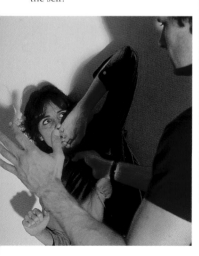

LEFT *Sometimes the startle pattern response is the only available response in an extraordinary situation.*

If your fight-or-flight reaction causes you to have a rigid retracted neck, then the muscles in the neck cannot operate normally. Ideally, the head-neck-back should be operating in a subtle free relationship, allowing lengthening in stature and widening to produce a posture in which optimum breathing is possible. When this relationship is upset, we become stiff, nervous, and tense.

"It is an interesting psychological fact that there are millions of educated people who have cultivated unwillingly the 'worry habit'. This unnecessary worry habit is directly the outcome of the lack of use of our reasoning faculties…"

Children can be seriously affected and the increase in childhood asthma, hypertension, heart attacks, and suicides gives sad evidence to the fact that the way we deal with stress in the psychophysical mechanism is having unacceptable effects. We long for *mens sana*

> The unexamined life is
> not worth living.
>
> **SOCRATES**

in corpore sano, "a sound mind in a sound body," a phrase that has been used for centuries to articulate an educational goal.

FIGHT OR FLIGHT

The short-term stress response called the fight-or-flight response exists to enable us to cope quickly with situations that are life-threatening. In these situations you need extra energy very quickly. The body deals with this need through biological changes. The pulse, blood pressure, and breathing rate all increase to boost energy. More blood is pumped through the blood vessels supplying the muscles, and the bronchial tubes dilate to allow extra air through with each breath. The palms of the hands and the soles of the feet start to perspire – a moist surface provides a better grip. The pupils of the eyes dilate to let in more light and improve vision. Reaction time speeds up.

This response is entirely normal and has probably saved our lives on many occasions. While it is perfectly normal to have this response, to maintain it for long periods is neurotic and unnecessary. When we are stressed we produce cortisol, a hormone that modifies how sensory information is processed in the body. In addition to this hormone, adrenalin is released. One of the quickest ways to reduce cortisol and adrenalin production is to have a good laugh. The biological changes that laughter produces are virtually the reverse of those that occur during a stress response.

The impact that stress has on you depends to a considerable degree upon the ability you have to control it. The Alexander Technique offers you a greater sense of personal control. Even if it were possible, we would not want to eliminate stress completely, as mild, brief, controllable stress can be stimulating and even enjoyable. A controlled amount of adrenalin can positively enhance performance.

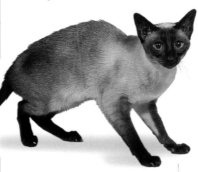

ABOVE *All animals use the fight-or-flight response as a means of survival. Humans tend to overmaintain the state.*

MALPOSTURE

The startle pattern may be taken as a paradigm of malposture in general, whether it is associated with aging, disease, or lack of exercise. In malposture, muscles in various combinations and degrees of tension have shortened, displacing the head or holding it in a fixed position. Head displacement would have an adverse effect on the rest of the body, partly because of the added weight and the strain put upon muscles and ligaments, but largely, I believe, because of interference in the righting reflexes by abnormal pressure on the joints of the neck. What is basically an incomplete response to gravity

would in time come to feel natural, and the muscles contributing to it would be strengthened by exercise.

Startle Pattern Reflex

In *Freedom to Change*, Frank Pierce Jones describes the startle reflex:

The pattern of startle is remarkably regular. It begins with an eye blink; the head is then thrust forward; the shoulders are raised and the arms stiffened; abdominal muscles shorten; breathing stops, and the knees are flexed. The pattern permits minor variations, but its primary features are the same. Because the startle response is brief and unexpected, it is difficult to observe and more difficult to control. Its chief interest here lies in the fact that it is the model of other, slower response patterns: fear, anxiety, fatigue, and pain all show postural changes from the norm that are similar to those that are seen in startle. In all of them, there is a shortening of neck muscles, which displaces the head, which is usually followed by some kind of flexion response, so that the body is drawn into a slightly smaller space. As in startle, these postural responses cannot take place without the prior displacement of the head and the shortening of the neck muscles. Since these responses are much slower than the startle response, they can be changed by controlling the first stage in the pattern, the head displacement, through which the rest of the pattern is propagated. Changing the response pattern simply means that the response will be rational and appropriate to the situation instead of an irrational stereotype.

> The body reflects the inner
> disposition of the mind.
>
> **ROBERT MACDONALD**

MAKING CHOICES

The Alexander Technique is about making choices in every aspect of your life, from how you behave to becoming the person you want to be. Alexander realized in the early stages of his experiments that he was unable to avoid his tendency to stiffen his neck and shorten his stature when he came to speak. He spent a long time observing himself in the mirror studying his behavior, and eventually he was able to adopt his full stature. However, when he began to recite again, he returned to his old pattern of stiffening and shortening. Alexander realized that the muscular pattern associated with speaking was deeply ingrained and that his new understanding of how to use his body in a free way was overridden by the old pattern. He was still unsuccessful at maintaining an efficient use of himself in the act of speaking. After all this time, his instincts continued to make the old response feel right and natural. So he was finally forced to adopt the following plan:

1 Inhibit any immediate response to the stimulus to speak the sentence.

2 Project in their sequence the directions for the primary control which I had reasoned out as being best for the purpose of bringing about the new and improved use of myself in speaking.

3 Continue to project these directions until I believed I was sufficiently familiar with them to employ them for the purpose of gaining my end and speaking the sentence.

4 While still continuing to project the directions for the new use I would stop and consciously reconsider my first decision and ask myself, "Shall I after all go on to gain the end I have decided upon and speak the sentence? Or shall I not? Or shall I go on to gain some other end altogether?," and then and there make a fresh decision, either:

a) not to gain my original end, in which case I would continue to project the directions for maintaining the new use and not go and

BELOW *Throughout our whole life, from childhood to old age, we are always making choices.*

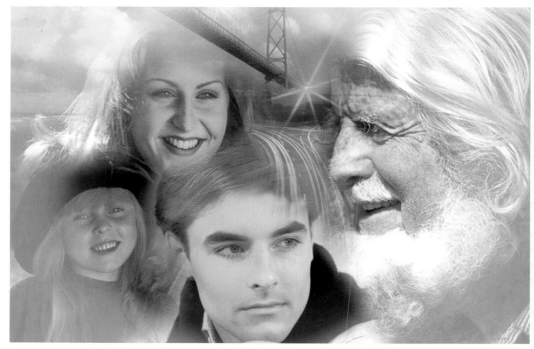

speak the sentence; or

b) to change my end and do something different, or to go on after all and gain my original end, in which case I would continue to project the directions for maintaining the new use to speak the sentence.

It was only when the conscious options to do, to not do, or to do something different existed up until the moment of action that Alexander overcame his instinctive misdirection. Many of us may find it difficult to break our habitual responses. When we examine our underlying motivation, we may find that we are being driven by the need to get it right, driven by our end-gaining tendency. Our commands to ourselves, however well-meaning, are immediately translated into the need to get it right. As long as we are fixed on getting things right, and getting it right now, we make it impossible for our organism, ourselves, to respond in a new way. We render ourselves inflexible. Our return to our habitual way of performing reflects our mental inflexibility. We assume that our bodies are the problem, but this is not the case. It is the mind that is in a muddle. We can only have choice when there are real alternatives to choose between. Once we have identified clear options in our mind, then the possibility of a new and different response becomes possible. We need to pay attention to the critical moment and practice working with it by becoming more conscious.

When we examine Alexander's method, we realize what the options that he put before himself opened up. Here is a chance for a new response that gives us insight into what it means to have the freedom to choose and in that learn to understand what it is to have free will.

The Readiness is All

The Alexander Technique helps you to build up the awareness that will help you to apply this strategy to your life. Think of any activity that is important to you, one in which you desire to be at your best and able to respond in the moment to the circumstances as they present themselves. Can you examine your situation in such a way that makes the three options relevant? Think about the alertness of mind that will be required in order to direct the use of yourselves and prepare in the way that Alexander did. Think of the detachment that will be required in order for you to be able to say "No" to your immediate response to the stimulus, and the alertness of mind that will be required to sustain that detachment throughout the situation. Think about the readiness of mind that will be required to make choices in the moment, and even to discover and be open to ones that you have not yet considered to be possible or achievable.

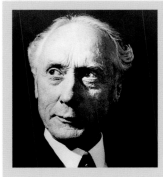
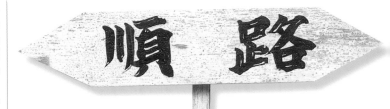

ABOVE *What do you think this sign says? The literal translation from Chinese is "This Way."*

Become Yourself

THE ALEXANDER TECHNIQUE *began with a man who, through solving his own problems, became able to help others realize that breath is life and life is breath. In the Bible, God made man of the dust of the ground, then breathed into his nostrils the breath of life, and he became a living soul. If you stop your breath, you will lose your life. We have a chance to make life easier for ourselves, not by dropping out or working harder but by becoming more aware and conscious. Being able to breathe fully allows you to be truly inspired.*

To Thine Own Self Be True

This way of achieving conscious control over yourself is the great gift of the Alexander Technique. It works wonderfully when you are unhappy, but it can be used through the day to monitor your state. You cannot expect to master it immediately, and you need to allow yourself to make mistakes. By beginning to appreciate what is possible, and dedicating yourself to the search for personal growth and development, you will unlock the blessing of your conscious mind.

Being Alive: The Unity of the Mind, Body, Spirit

The division of the mind and body is absolutely false. The Alexander Technique helps you to become more conscious of the subtle but critical interactions between the mind and body. As your awareness of posture improves, your ability to feel what is happening in your body increases and you can become more sensitive to the disharmony that occurs in your nervous system as a result of internal and external pressure. From this comes the possibility of avoiding and dealing with stress,

> Our remedies oft in ourselves
> do lie
>
> **WILLIAM SHAKESPEARE:**
> *ALLS WELL THAT ENDS WELL*

heightening your resistance to disease, registering a latent disposition before it turns into overt disease and accelerating the healing process when you have become ill.

Taking Charge of Yourself

Whether we like it or not, the self is always oriented in a particular direction. We may refuse to admit or to pay attention to what our direction is, but we are always in a state of mind and making a decision to remain in that state or to not. Even idleness is a direction – it is the direction of not moving.

Sometimes our direction is positive – we are up, energized, at one with ourselves, making conscious choices and in charge of our direction. At other times we are down, depressed, lacking in optimism, overwhelmed by negative emotions

> The Kingdom is
> inside you
> and it is outside you
> When you come to
> know yourselves
> Then you will
> become known
>
> **GOSPEL OF THOMAS**
> **CE 150 FOUND IN 1945**
> **IN EGYPT**

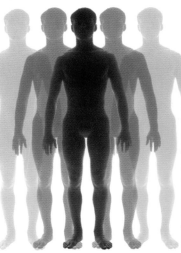

BELOW *By using your conscious mind, you can begin to come into focus.*

such as bitterness, feelings of inadequacy, or jealousy. These feelings often create more conflict because one half of the self wants to be positive, and when we find ourselves responding negatively, we get negative about being negative, and the whole situation gets compounded and we find ourselves in a vicious downward spiral. But, nevertheless, we are choosing. The Alexander Technique is a powerful strategy that can help us learn to deal with our negative patterns.

Achieving your full potential

There is an old Sufi tale that tells of our search for answers. After the gods had created the world, they decided they would create truth. In order that we humans should not discover it immediately, they decided to hide truth. Should it be put on the highest mountain, or in the deepest cave? The oldest and wisest god had the best idea. He suggested hiding truth in the very heart of us, knowing that we would look all over the world long before we thought to look inside ourselves.

Getting to know ourselves and finding our way are becoming very important to more and more people today. We no longer blame circumstances, birth, or even luck. We are coming to realize that it is we who are the instigators and solvers of our problems. Of course, things happen in our lives that cause us pain and heartache, and we wonder what we have done to be in such a situation. Once we realize that we can help ourselves, we begin to understand and use some proven ways to gain the ends we want.

> What a piece of work is a man!
> How noble in reason! How
> infinite is faculty! in form, in
> moving, how express and
> admirable! In action how like an
> angel! In apprehension how like a
> god! The beauty of the world!
> The paragon of animals.
>
> **WILLIAM SHAKESPEARE,**
> **HAMLET**

The Alexander Technique is a practical way that we can begin this process, by helping us to recognize and eventually prevent the habits that hold us back. Through an understanding of conscious inhibition and conscious direction, we can give ourselves more time and space in our daily lives. We can begin to come into our true inheritance. Hamlet gave us the words; we now have the opportunity to fulfill them.

STRATEGY FOR CHANGE

1 Stop. Give yourself time and practice conscious inhibition.
2 Accept how you are feeling. Open your eyes to the situation as it is now and take responsibility for it.
3 Be aware of your head, neck, and back, and your breathing pattern. Notice the relationship between your postural aspect, your emotional responses, and your thought patterns. Let your sensory appreciation inform you of the state of your muscles.
4 Ask, "Is this the state in which I want to be?"
5 If the answer is "Yes," then that is what you have chosen.
6 If the answer is "No," then you can choose to change by allowing your neck to be free so your head can go forward and your back can lengthen and widen. Breathe out, then allow the air to return fully, quickly, and freely.

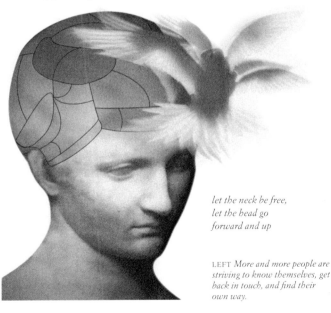

*let the neck be free,
let the head go
forward and up*

LEFT *More and more people are
striving to know themselves, get
back in touch, and find their
own way.*

Further Reading/Useful Addresses

ALEXANDER, F.M., *Articles and Lectures* Compiled by Jean M.O. Fischer, Mouritz, London, 1995.

ALEXANDER, F.M., *Conscious Constructive Control of the Individual*, STAT Books, London 1997.

ALEXANDER, F.M., *Man's Supreme Inheritance,* Mouritz, London, 1996.

ALEXANDER, F.M., *The Universal Constant in Living,* Mouritz, London, 2000.

BARLOW, W., *The Alexander Principle,* London, Gollancz, 1973.

BINKLEY, G., *The Expanding Self,* Edited by Jean M. O. Fischer. STAT Books, London, 1993.

BROWN, R., *Authorized Summaries of F: M. Alexander's Four Books,* STAT Books, London, 1992.

CAPLAN, D., *Back Trouble,* Triad Publishing Co., Gainsville, Florida, 1987.

Acknowledgments

Picture credits:
CAMERON COLLECTION:*pp 20t*
CORBIS/STOCKMARKET: *pps 36l, 134, 135*
THE GLOBE THEATRE, LONDON: *pp 92b*
GETTYONE/FPG INTERNATIONAL: *pp 104b*
GETTYONE/STONE: *pp 110t*
NASA: *pp 36r*
(t:top; b: bottom; l: left; r: right)

Authors Acknowledgments:
I wish to thank all my fellow Alexander Teachers who contributed their knowledge: Peri Aston, Malcolm Balk, Jean Clark, Katerina Diss, Helene Corrie, Pedro de Alcantara, Graham Griffiths, H. Hatada, Roger Kidd, Felicity Lipman, Ilana Machover, Gordon McCaffrey, Tessa Marwick, Sue Merry, Tess Miller, Daniel Pevsner, Joe Searby, Lori Schiff, Judy Stern, Steven Shaw, Frank Trembath, M. Wohl; and all my students. Finally as Shakespeare said, "Thanks, thanks and ever thanks" to Walter and Dilys Carrington, my husband Robert, and children Jessie and Jack.

CARRINGTON, W., and Carey, S., *Explaining the Alexander Technique: The Writings of F: Matthias Alexander.* The Sheildrake Press, London, 1992.

DART, RAYMOND A., *Skill and Poise.* STAT Books, London, 1996.

DE ALCANTARA, P., *Indirect Procedures: A Musicians Guide to the Alexander Technique,* Oxford University Press, Oxford, 1997.

EVANS, JACKIE, *Frederick Matthais Alexander, A Family History,* Phillimore, 2001.

GARLICK, DAVID. *The Lost Sixth Sense, A Medical Scientist Looks at the Alexander Technique.* University of New South Wales, Kensington, 1990.

JONES, F.P., *Freedom to Change: The Development and Science of the Alexander Technique,* Mouritz, London, 1997.

LANGFORD E., *Mind and Muscle, An Owner's Handbook,* Garant, 1999.

LEIBOWITZ, J., CONNINGTON, B., *The Alexander Technique,* Harper and Row, 1990.

MACDONALD, ROBERT., *The Use of the Voice: Sensory Appreciation, Posture, Vocal Functioning and Shakespearean Text Performance.* Macdonald Media, London, 1997.

MACDONALD, ROBERT & NESS CARO, *Secrets of the Alexander Technique* Dorling Kindersley, 2001

MACDONALD, ROBERT, *The Voice Handbook* Macdonald Media, 2001

SHAW, S., AND D'ANGOUR, A., *The Art of Swimming,* Ashgrove Press Limited, Bath, 1996.

Institutions Using the Alexander Technique

UK

The Royal Shakespeare Company, Shakespeare's Globe, London, the London Academy of Music and Dramatic Art, the Royal Academy of Dramatic Art, the Guildhall School of Music and Drama, the Royal National Theatre, the Central School of Speech and Drama, Guildford Drama School, Mountview Theatre School, the Royal Academy of Music, the Royal College of Music, the Royal Northern College of Music and the Purcell School, London Academy of Theater.

USA

The Juilliard School New York University, Mannes College of Music, The Actor's Studio, The American Academy of Dramatic Arts. Northwestern University School of Music and School of Speech, Yale University, The Aspen Music Festival and School, New England Conservatory of Music, The Eastman School of Music, American Conservatory Theatre, San Francisco, Boston University

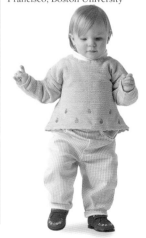

Australia – AUSTAT
PO Box 716
Darlinghurst
NSW 2010
Tel: +61 (0)2 9247 5991
www.alexandertechnique.org.au

Belgium – AEFMAT
4 Rue des Fonds
B-1380 Lasne
Tel: +32 2633 3059
Fax: +32 2633 3059
www.fmalexandertech.be

Brazil – ABTA
Caixa Postal 16020
Rio de Janeiro
RJ Brasil
CEP 22220-970
Tel: +55 21 239 666 18
Fax: +55 21 239 66 18
www.geocities.com/abta.geo

Canada – CANSTAT
Howerd Brockner
465 Wilson Avenue
Toronto
Ontario
Canada
M3H 1TP
Tel: +1 416 631 8127
Fax: +1 416 631 0094
www.canstat.ca

Denmark– DFLAT
Lis Jakobsen
Gasse 5, Gl. Holte
DK 2840 Holte
Tel: +45 7025 5070

France – L'Association Française des
Professeurs de la Technique Alexander
(APTA)
Paola d'Alba
42 Terrasse de l'Iris
La Defence 2
92400 Courbevoire
France

Tel: +33 1 4090 0623
Fax: +33 1 4090 0623
www.perso.wanadoo.fr/technique.
alexander

Germany – GLAT
Postfach 5312
79020
Freiburg
Tel: +49 761 38 33 57
Fax: +49 761 38 33 57
www.alexander.technik.org

Israel – ISTAT
PO Box 16163
Tel Aviv 61161
Tel: +972 522 7979

Netherlands – NeVLAT
Postbus 15591
1001 NB Amsterdam
Tel: +31 206 253 163

New Zealand – Alexander Technique
Teachers Society
New Zealand (ATTSNZ)
PO Box 3020
Wellington
New Zealand

South Africa – South African Society of
Teachers of the Alexander Technique
(SASTAT)
PO Box 135
Simon's Town 7995
South Africa
Tel: +27 21 780 9412

Spain – Asociación de Profesores de la
Technica (APTAE)
Tel: +34 91532 01 05
Fax: +34 9152358 17
www.teleline.terra.es/personal/fmalexan
der/sp

Switzerland – (SVLAT)
Postfach 8032
Zurich
Tel: +41 (0)1 201 03 43

United Kingdom – Society for the
Teachers of the Alexander Technique
(STAT)
129 Camden Mews
London NW1 9AH
Tel: +44 (020) 7284 3338
Fax: +44 (020) 7284 5435
www.stat.org.uk

London – London Academy of Theater
LLC
9 Mason's Island Road
Mystic CT 06355
Tel/Fax (020) 860 245 3632
www.londonacedemyoftheater.edu

Macdonald Media Ltd
www.macdonaldmedia.co.uk

The London Academy of Music and
Dramatic Art
266 Cromwell Road
London
SW5 0SR
Tel: +44 (020) 7373 9883
www.lamda.org.uk

Shakespeare's Globe
21 New Globe Walk
Bankside
London
SE1 9DT
Tel: +44 (020) 7902 1400
Fax: + 44 (020) 7902 1401
www.shakespeare-globe.org

USA – The American Society for the
Alexander Technique (AmSAT)
PO Box 60008
Florence
MA 01062
Tel: + (413) 584 2359
Fax: : (413) 584 3097
www.alexandertech.org

The Julliard School
60 Lincoln Center Plaza
New York City
NY 10023
Tel: (1) 212 799 5000

Glossary

Action potential: Electrical energy generated by nerve or muscle activity.

Anatomical position: The body standing erect, face forward, arms at the side and palms forward.

Anoxia: Oxygen deprivation.

Antagonist: A muscle that acts in opposition to another.

Anterior: Toward the front,

Appendicular skeleton: The skeleton of the extremities and of the pectoral and pelvic girdles.

Artho-: Pertaining to a joint.

Arthrodia: A joint permitting only gliding movements.

Axial skeleton: The skeleton of the head and trunk.

Bilateral: Pertaining to both sides.

Cartilage: A nonvascular connective tissue, more flexible than bone.

Cell: The smallest unit of life. Contains a nucleus, protoplasm, and a cell wall.

Circumduction: When the end of a limb describes a circle, and the shaft escribes a cone.

Congenital: Existing at birth. May or may not be hereditary.

Conscious control: The natural faculty that enables us to organize our responses and reflexes in a directed and disciplined way.

Cortex: The outer layer of an organ.

Diaphragm: The dome-shaped muscle which separates the chest cavity from the abdominal cavity.

Directions: The process involved in projecting messages from the brain to the body mechanism to release, lengthen, and widen.

Enarthrodial: A joint in which a rounded head fits into a socket of another. Ball and socket.

End-gaining: Trying to achieve an end-result without adequate thought about how the movement is performed, which often leads to uncoordinated activity.

Extension: To increase the angle between bones.

Exteroceptor: Specialized sense organs that respond to pressure, temperature, and pain. The nerve endings are on the surface of the body.

Flexion: Decrease the angle between bones.

Ganglion: A mass of nerve cells located outside the central nervous system.

Hyperkinesia: Excessive movement.

Impulse: A stimulus carried by the nervous system.

Inhibition: (1) The learned faculty that allows time to consider how an action is to be performed before proceeding. (2) Essential neurological process.

Innervation: The supplying of any organ with nerve fibers.

Insertion: The area of attachment of a muscle to the bone it moves.

Intervertebral: That space between the vertebrae.

Kinaesthesia: The sense of movement of muscles, and the perception of weight, resistance, and position.

Lateral: Toward the side.

Ligament: A band of flexible, elastic, dense, fibrous connective tissue connecting the articular ends of bones.

Lumbar: Pertaining to the loin.

Means whereby: The thought given to how an action is achieved.

Membrane: A layer of tissue that binds structures, separates or lines cavities.

Opposition: Moving the thumb to touch the tips of the fingers.

Origin: The place of attachment of a muscle which remains fixed during contraction.

Pathology: A biological science dealing with the nature of disease, its courses, and its effects.

Pectoral: Pertaining to the chest.

Pelvis: A basin or basin-shaped cavity.

Physiology: The science of the function of living organisms, or their parts.

Primary control: The balance of the head in relation to the neck and back.

Prime mover: Muscle responsible for producing a particular movement.

Proprioception: The sense of position or movement of one part of the body relative to another.

Proprioceptor: Receptor located in the muscles, tendons and joints, which allows the body to recognize its position.

Reflex: An involuntary, relatively invariable adaptive response to a stimulus.

Somatic: Pertaining to the body and especially the voluntary muscles and skeletal framework.

Stature: The total natural height from the soles of the feet to the crown of the head.

Supine: Lying on the back, face upward, or the hand with palm upward.

Synovial: Pertaining to the secretion of synovial fluid by the membranes in an articular capsule.

Tendon: A non-elastic band of connective tissue which forms the attachment of muscle to bone.

Tensor: That part of a muscle which serves to make a structure tense.

Tissue: An aggregate of cells similar in function.

Index